Simple Treatments
for Complex Problems

*A Flexible Cognitive Behavior Analysis
System Approach to Psychotherapy*

Simple Treatments for Complex Problems

A Flexible Cognitive Behavior Analysis System Approach to Psychotherapy

Kimberly A. Driscoll
Kelly C. Cukrowicz
Maureen Lyons Reardon
Thomas E. Joiner, Jr.
The Florida State University

In collaboration with the staff of
The Florida State University Psychology Clinic

Ginette C. Blackhart	Jennifer A. Minnix
Leonardo Bobadilla	Marisol Perez
Andrea B. Burns	Scharles C. Petty
Keith F. Donohue	Mark D. Reeves
Rebecca R. Gerhardstein	Lorraine R. Reitzel
Annya Hernandez	Karla K. Repper
Therese Skubic Kemper	Sarah A. Shultz
Donald R. Kerr, Jr.	Sheila L. Stanley
Rita L. Ketterman	Bradley A. White

Copyright © 2004 by Lawrence Erlbaum Associates, Inc.
All rights reserved.

No part of this book may be reproduced in any form,
by photostat, microfilm, retrieval system, or any other means,
without prior written permission of the publisher.
    Lawrence Erlbaum Associates, Inc., Publishers
    10 Industrial Avenue
    Mahwah, NJ 07430

Cover design by Kathryn Houghtaling Lacey

Library of Congress Cataloging-in-Publication Data

Simple treatments for complex problems : a flexible cognitive behavior
analysis system approach to psychotherapy / Kimberly A. Driscoll . . . [et al.]
in collaboration with the staff of the Florida State University Psychology Clinic.
    p. cm.
    Includes bibliographical references and indexes.
    ISBN 0–8058–4643–3 (cloth : alk. paper)
    1. Cognitive therapy. I. Driscoll, Kimberly A., 1972–   II. Florida State
University. Psychology Clinic.

RC489.C63S565 2004
616.89'14—dc22   2003049294

10 9 8 7 6 5 4 3 2

Contents

About the Authors		vii
Preface		ix
Chapter 1	The Cognitive Behavioral Analysis System of Psychotherapy: Modifications and Applications for a Variety of Psychological Disorders	1

PART I Personality Disorders

Chapter 2	Schizotypal Personality Disorder	15
Chapter 3	Borderline Personality Disorder	33
Chapter 4	Passive-Aggressive (Negativistic) Personality Disorder	49
Chapter 5	Personality Disorder Not Otherwise Specified	67

PART II Anxiety Disorders

Chapter 6	Social Anxiety Disorder and Avoidant Personality Disorder	81
Chapter 7	Generalized Anxiety Disorder and Panic Disorder	101

PART III Parents, Children, and Couples

Chapter 8	Parents of Children Diagnosed With Behavior Disorders	119
Chapter 9	Children With Social Skills Deficits	139
Chapter 10	Couples	153

PART IV Other Issues and Groups

Chapter 11	Anger Management Problems	169

| Chapter 12 | Correctional Settings | 187 |
| Chapter 13 | The Cognitive Behavioral Analysis System of Psychotherapy: Future Directions | 207 |

References	225
Author Index	235
Subject Index	239

About the Authors

Kimberly A. Driscoll, Kelly C. Cukrowicz, and Maureen Lyons Reardon are doctoral candidates in clinical psychology at Florida State University, where Thomas E. Joiner is the Bright-Burton Professor of Psychology and Director of the University Psychology Clinic.

Driscoll's work has focused on childhood depression, the assessment of ADHD and child externalizing disorders, and adherence in children with type 1 diabetes; Cukrowicz's, on predictors of treatment outcome, evaluation of prevention methods for anxiety and depression, and adult and child psychopathology; Reardon's on substance use and schizophrenia, mechanisms underlying acute alcohol tolerance, substance use in special populations (e.g., correctional institutions, homeless), evaluations of competency/criminal responsibility, and predictors of psychotherapy outcome. Joiner's interests include the psychology and neurobiology of depression, suicidal behavior, anxiety, and eating disorders. He earned a PhD in clinical psychology at the University of Texas at Austin. A recipient of a Guggenheim Fellowship and the American Psychological Association Distinguished Scientific Award for Early Career Contribution to Psychology in the area of psychopathology, among other awards, he is the coauthor or editor of six books and the author of more than 200 journal articles and chapters. He has also served as Associate Editor of *Behavior Therapy* and as a member of the editorial boards of nine other journals.

Preface

The primary goal of psychotherapy is to help patients get better. As a result of managed care and limitations set forth by insurance companies, it has become increasingly important for therapists to quickly facilitate the patient's process of getting better. Thus, there has been a movement toward developing psychological treatments that can be easily and efficiently implemented. Moreover, it is incumbent on therapists to provide patients with treatments that work. McCullough (2000) developed such a treatment; his Cognitive Behavioral Analysis System of Psychotherapy (CBASP) is a technique that has proven to be efficacious in the treatment of chronic depression. In addition, the highly structured nature of the technique allows for ease of learning and implementation. The underlying concept of CBASP is simple. The therapist assists the patient in discovering why he or she did not obtain a Desired Outcome (DO) by evaluating the patient's problematic thoughts and behaviors. In other words, the therapist helps the patient to determine what thoughts and behaviors got in the way of getting a DO. Because there is often a mismatch between a patient's goals and what is actually happening in the patient's life, CBASP's technique can easily be adapted and used in the treatment of other psychologically distressing problems, including anxiety, personality disorders, marital conflict, and child behavior problems.

Simple Treatments for Complex Problems: A Flexible Cognitive Behavior Analysis System Approach to Psychotherapy demonstrates the wider application of CBASP to a variety of psychological disorders. Furthermore, the chapters in this book provide clinicians and patients with valuable information regarding the implementation and modification of CBASP through abundant clinical case examples and in-session transcripts.[1] This book should prove valuable to academicians, researchers, clinicians, other

---

[1] All names in case examples were changed to protect patients' identity.

service providers, and the general public, particularly those interested in conducting treatment research and those interested in providing or receiving efficient and effective treatment. CBASP, as presented in this book, is simple to teach and implement and provides both professionals and the general public with an efficient and effective means to improve psychological functioning.

The idea for this book was suggested by the director of the Florida State University (FSU) Psychology Clinic, Thomas E. Joiner, PhD. One morning during our weekly staff meeting, Dr. Joiner stated that it would be a good idea for someone to write a book applying McCullough's CBASP technique to other psychological disorders. As the assistant director at the time, I gave Dr. Joiner's idea some thought and then asked him if we as a clinic could write the book, especially since we used CBASP to treat a variety of disorders. At first he was skeptical; he was not convinced that the therapists would be enthusiastic about joining him in writing a book given that they already had multiple clinical-related, research-related, and course-related responsibilities. Despite the amount of work that the project represented, all of us were enthusiastic, and as a result this book is a rather unique contribution to the field. Not only does it describe how to apply a single innovative and effective psychological treatment to a variety of psychological disorders, it was the product of a collaborative writing effort by the therapists at the FSU Psychology Clinic. As one of the coordinating authors (and I speak for the others and for all of the contributing authors), I am extremely grateful for Dr. Joiner's generosity and mentorship at the clinic, which has resulted in the acquisition of what we feel are superior clinical and research skills by us, his mentees and in what we hope will be a widely influential and widely used treatment technique that will help patients get better fast.

— *Kimberly A. Driscoll*

Chapter 1

The Cognitive Behavioral Analysis System of Psychotherapy: Modifications and Applications for a Variety of Psychological Disorders*

> The introduction will provide a comprehensive review of the disorders that are discussed in subsequent chapters. In addition, the Cognitive Behavioral Analysis System of Psychotherapy will be described, and general guidelines for modifications are proposed.

Recently, there has been a movement away from the traditional approach to psychotherapy (a patient sitting on a couch as the therapist makes interpretations connecting the past to the present) to a more time-limited, goal-directed approach, with a particular emphasis on the present. This movement toward the more efficient delivery of psychotherapy serves several purposes. First, it helps patients recover in a shorter amount of time, which has implications for decreasing the negative impact of psychological distress in a variety of areas, including interpersonal relationships, employment, and personal finance. Second, it decreases the cost of psychotherapy while at the same time potentially increasing the number of patients who receive services. Finally, as researchers and clinicians continue to refine and

---

*The primary authors contributing to this chapter were Kimberly A. Driscoll, Kelly C. Cukrowicz, and Thomas E. Joiner, Jr.

improve psychotherapeutic techniques, it reinforces the scientific bases of psychotherapy and enhances credibility.

The movement has resulted in the establishment of a variety of treatments as efficacious (i.e., shown to work for a group of patients with a specific psychological disorder under well controlled conditions). For example, the current treatment of choice for a patient diagnosed with obsessive-compulsive disorder is the combination of pharmacotherapy with exposure and response prevention. In some cases, there exists more than one empirically supported treatment for a specific psychological disorder (see Chambless & Ollendick, 2000, for a complete review of currently empirically supported therapies). Many different therapeutic techniques have been demonstrated to be equally efficacious for depression. For example, improvement in functioning is seen in depressed patients whether the primary treatment modality is pharmacotherapy, psychotherapy, or a combination of the two.

Recently, Keller et al. (2000) demonstrated that the Cognitive Behavioral Analysis System of Psychotherapy (CBASP), particularly in combination with pharmacotherapy, is efficacious in the treatment of chronic depression. CBASP is goal oriented, efficient, and simple to implement.

THE DEVELOPMENT OF CBASP

McCullough (2000) developed CBASP specifically for the treatment of chronic depression. The approach combines behavioral, cognitive, and interpersonal techniques to teach the patient to focus on the consequences of behavior, and to use problem solving to resolve interpersonal difficulties. The study that launched CBASP as an efficacious treatment took place at 12 academic centers and included patients who met criteria for a chronic unipolar depressive disorder (i.e., Major Depressive Disorder, recurrent or Dysthymic Disorder). Patients were randomly assigned to one of three treatment groups: medication only (Nefazodone), psychotherapy only (CBASP), or combined treatment of Nefazodone and CBASP. Extreme care was taken to ensure the qualifications and training of the therapists administering psychotherapy. In addition, treatment fidelity was carefully monitored and controlled. Results indicated that patients in all three treatment groups improved substantially. However, those patients who received the combined treatment of Nefazodone and CBASP made even more significant improvements on posttreatment ratings, compared with those patients in either the medication-only treatment

COMPONENTS OF CBASP

group or the psychotherapy-only treatment group. Thus, the authors concluded that their results contribute to the extant literature, suggesting that the combination of medication and psychotherapy in the treatment of depression is superior to either treatment alone.

COMPONENTS OF CBASP

The primary exercise of CBASP is Situational Analysis, or SA, in which there is an elicitation phase and a remediation phase (McCullough, 2000). SA first requires the patient to verbalize his or her contribution in a distressful situation at three levels: interpersonally, behaviorally, and cognitively. SA is accomplished in five steps: describing the situation, stating the interpretations that were made during the situation, describing the behaviors that occurred, stating the desired outcome, and stating the actual outcome. When first beginning CBASP, the Coping Survey Questionnaire (CSQ)[1] should be used both in session and as assigned homework (see Fig. 1.1). The CSQ is introduced in the first session as the tool with which CBASP is conducted. The overall goal of the treatment is to determine the discrepancy between what the patient wants to happen in a specific situation and what is actually happening. By examining the specific situations, the patient gradually uncovers problematic themes and ways in which he or she can get what is wanted.

The patient is told that he or she will complete CSQs about stressful or problematic interactions. The patient is also told that the situation will be discussed in session, along with what the patient thought, how he or she acted, and how the situation turned out compared with how the patient wanted the situation to turn out. Finally, the patient is told that this method will allow him or her to determine ways in which thoughts and behaviors are interfering with his or her ability to get the desired outcome.

As noted, the CSQ is the primary tool of SA, and we have made modifications to McCullough's original CSQ to facilitate the efficient use of this important tool, which is reflected in the descriptions of each of the steps. The CSQ is introduced in the first session. Providing the patient with several blank copies of the CSQ establishes the expectation that at least two CSQs are to be completed between sessions, which means at least one CSQ

---

[1] We recommend several modifications to McCullough's CSQ; therefore, we refer to our version as the Coping Survey Questionnaire Used in the FSU Psychology Clinic's Adaptations of CBASP.

> **Coping Survey Questionnaire**
> **Used in FSU Psychology Clinic's**
> **Adaptations of CBASP**
>
> Select a stressful situation that has occurred in your life during the previous
> week or two. Please describe this situation using the steps indicated below.
>
> 1. In three or four sentences, describe the situation.
>
> 2. What was your interpretation of the situation? What did this situation
>   mean to you?
>   a.
>   b.
>   c.
>   d.
>
> 3. What were your behaviors in this situation?
>   a. Eye Contact—
>   b. Body Posture—
>   c. Gestures—
>   d. Tone of Voice—
>   e. Timing—
>   f. Other behaviors—
>
>   What did you say? How did you say it?
>
> 4. State what you wanted to get out of this situation. What was your desired
>   outcome?
>
> 5. What was the actual outcome of this situation?
>
> **RATE:** Did you get what you wanted? Yes _____ No _____

FIG. 1.1. Coping Survey Questionnaire used in Situational Analysis. Adapted from McCullough's Coping Survey Questionnaire by Maureen Lyons Reardon.

will be reviewed in session. Initially, completing one CSQ will probably take a full session; however, as the patient becomes more succinct when completing the individual steps and more efficient with using the CSQ, it is likely that several CSQs can be completed in one session. Eventual mastery of the steps of the CSQ is expected; however, patients should be required to complete a paper version of the CSQ as homework between every session to ensure consolidation of therapeutic gains. A graphical depiction of the CSQ can be found in Fig. 1.2, which can also be used as a patient handout to explain the process.

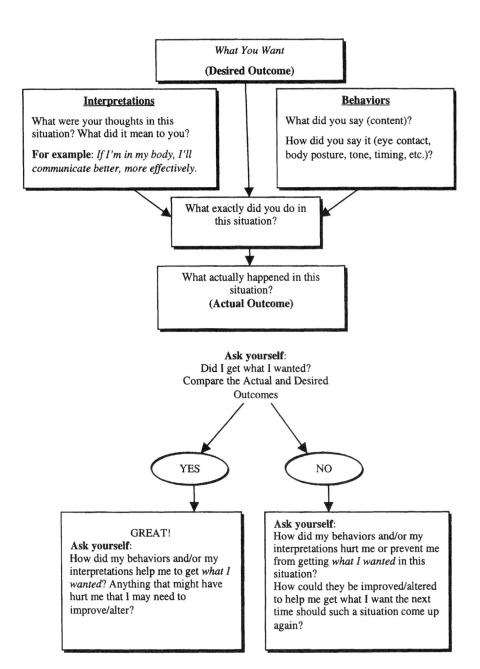

FIG. 1.2. Graphical depiction of CSQ format used to facilitate discussion of the connections between thoughts, behaviors, and consequent outcomes. Adapted by Maureen Lyons Reardon.

In Step 1, the patient succinctly describes a problematic or stressful situation in an objective manner. The goal during this step is for the patient to provide a situation with a beginning, a middle, and an end, without editorializing or making interpretations about what happened. We refer to this as a specific slice of time, and our goal is for patients to describe very specific situations. The therapist may phrase the elicitation of Step 1 as "If I was a fly on the wall, what would I see?" The information presented in Step 1 needs to be both relevant and accurate. Because patients often provide irrelevant, extraneous information, instructing the patient to describe a discrete incident in three or four sentences is recommended.

During Step 2, the patient learns to identify the specific interpretations that were made during the situation. Depression-related interpretations tend to be global and negative in nature. The goal of the second step is for the patient to construct relevant and accurate interpretations, and the most effective interpretations are those that contribute directly to the attainment of the Desired Outcome (DO). This step tends to be the most difficult for patients to complete; thus, instructing them to describe two or three thoughts that popped into their mind often helps with identifying interpretations. Sometimes it is necessary for the therapist to prompt the patient by stating, "At the time, when you were in the situation, what did it mean to you?"

During Step 3 of SA, the patient identifies the specific behaviors that occurred during the situation. Particular attention is paid to the content of the conversation, the tone of voice, body language, eye contact, and anything else that the patient did (e.g., walking away). When identifying behaviors, the patient should attempt to use the tone of voice or facial expressions that occurred in the situation so that the behavioral details are accurately replicated. The goal of Step 3 is for the patient to focus on the aspects of his or her behavior that contribute to the attainment of the DO.

Identification of the DO is accomplished in Step 4.[2] Articulating the DO is important because all steps are anchored or related to the attainment of the DO. The DO is the outcome that the patient actually wanted in the given situation. To facilitate the expression of the DO the therapist can ask, "What were you trying to get in this situation?" or "How did you want this

---

[2] It should be noted that in McCullough's (2000) original conceptualization of CBASP Steps 4 and 5 are reversed; the AO is determined in Step 4 and the DO is determined in Step 5. However, given that all steps are anchored to the DO, it is the opinion of these authors that the DO should be emphasized before discussion of the AO. Therefore, these steps have been reordered throughout the remaining chapters.

1. COGNITIVE BEHAVIORAL ANALYSIS SYSTEM

situation to turn out?" It is important for the patient to identify a single DO per CSQ. Moreover, the patient's goal in Step 4 is to construct DOs that are attainable and realistic, meaning that the outcome can be produced by the environment and the patient has the capacity to produce the outcome. Patients often have difficulty determining the appropriate DO because they begin by choosing an outcome that requires change in another person or a change in their emotions. The patient must always focus on how his or her own thoughts and behaviors influence situations, and, when focusing on how someone else reacts, the patient should be reminded that others can be influenced but not controlled.

Lastly, the identification of the Actual Outcome (AO) is accomplished in Step 5. The patient's goal during Step 5 is to construct an AO using behavioral terminology that describes exactly what happened in the situation. Patients usually do not have any difficulty stating the AO; however, for patients who have difficulty articulating this step, asking the question "What did you really get?" might help. Once Steps 1 through 5 are complete, the patient compares the AO to the DO, answering the most important question—whether or not he or she got the DO. This completes the elicitation phase.

During the remediation phase, behaviors and cognitions are targeted for change and revised so that the patient's new behaviors and cognitions in the situation contribute to the DO. Thus, during the remediation phase, each interpretation is assessed to determine whether it aided in or hindered the attainment of the DO. The remediation step focused on behaviors is similar to that done in the remediation step focused on interpretation: Each behavior is evaluated as to whether or not the behavior aided in or hindered the attainment of the DO.

If interpretations or behaviors are seen as obstacles to attainment of DOs, the solution is simply to alter them so the interpretations or behaviors are more likely to lead to DOs. Repetition of these steps in a variety of specific life situations is the core of the CBASP technique (McCullough, 2000).

APPLICATION OF CBASP TO OTHER PSYCHOLOGICAL DISORDERS

Although McCullough (2000) originally developed CBASP for patients with chronic depression, the general principles of CBASP can be applied to a variety of psychological disorders, and in some cases only minimal modifications to the original technique are necessary. As noted previously, the primary exercise of CBASP is SA, in which there is an elicitation phase and a remediation phase. This is accomplished using the CSQ. SA first requires patients to verbalize their contribution in a social encounter at three levels: interpersonally, behaviorally, and cognitively. During the remediation phase, behaviors and cognitions are targeted for change and revised so that the patients' new behaviors and cognitions in the situation contribute to a desirable outcome. Because most psychological disorders result in some form of interpersonal difficulty, the use of SA across a variety of disorders makes intuitive sense. For example, patients with personality disorders undoubtedly have interpersonal conflicts, patients with social anxiety disorder may experience such extreme anxiety when conversing with others that the possibility of forming and fostering relationships is impaired, and patients with impulse control disorders, particularly anger management problems, may alienate others to the point that the relationship is left in ruins. Thus, SA via the CSQ can be used to address one of the common features in each of these disorders—interpersonal difficulties.

Personality Disorders

A personality disorder is defined as an enduring pattern of thinking, feeling, and behaving that markedly deviates from the expectations of one's culture (American Psychiatric Association, 1994). This pattern of experience and behavior is pervasive, inflexible, and stable over time and leads to significant distress or impairment in the individual. There are three clusters of personality disorders. Cluster A consists of paranoid, schizoid, and schizotypal personality disorders; individuals diagnosed with a personality disorder in this category are often described as odd and eccentric. Cluster B consists of antisocial, borderline, histrionic, and narcissistic personality disorders; individuals diagnosed with a personality disorder in this category are described as dramatic or erratic. Finally, Cluster C consists of avoidant, dependent, and obsessive-compulsive personality disorders; individuals diagnosed with these disorders often appear anxious or fearful. Relatively few treatments have been determined to be efficacious for personality disorders. In fact, according to Nathan and Gorman (1998), there are standard psychosocial treatments for Borderline Personality Disorder (BPD) and Avoidant Personality Disorder (APD) but none for other personality disorders.

The application of CBASP to personality disorders is described in Chapters 2 through 5, which cover Schizotypal Personality Disorder (STPD), BPD, Passive-Aggressive Personality Disorder (PAPD), and Personality Disorder Not Otherwise Specified (PD NOS). STPD is characterized by a pattern of maladaptive interpersonal behavior and by specific cognitive and behavioral symptoms (e.g., stereotyped thinking, magical thinking, odd/eccentric demeanor, tangential speech). Previous studies indicate this disorder can be successfully treated with cognitive behavioral therapy. Chapter 2 describes modifications of CBASP that apply the use of this technique to STPD.

BPD consists of symptoms such as instability of interpersonal relationships, self-image, and affect and a pattern of marked impulsivity. This disorder traditionally has been considered among the more difficult to treat, in part due to the interpersonal deficits these patients exhibit. Chapter 3 summarizes the application of CBASP to BPD and suggests ways in which it complements existing treatments for the disorder.

PAPD is described in Chapter 4. The disorder is characterized by a pattern of negativistic attitudes, passive resistance to the demands of others, and negative reactivity (e.g., hostile defiance, scorning of authority). This disorder is currently described in the appendix of the *Diagnostic and Statistical Manual of Mental Disorders–Fourth Edition* (*DSM–IV;* American Psychiatric Association, 1994), as a result of controversy surrounding the validity of the diagnosis. There is currently no empirically validated treatment for this disorder; however, CBASP seems to be a promising new frontier in reducing the attitudes and behaviors associated with PAPD.

PD NOS is the diagnostic label applied to patients who present with a combination of pathological personality symptoms that comprise the other personality disorders but do not present with symptoms that meet the full criteria for any one personality disorder. These symptoms may also include more than one personality disorder cluster (i.e., odd/eccentric, anxious, or dramatic/erratic). Chapter 5 presents CBASP as a method of treating the multifaceted presentations that make up this disorder. A case example describes the implementation of SA for a patient with PD NOS with avoidant and schizotypal features.

Anxiety Disorders

Anxiety disorders are the most heterogeneous of all the diagnostic categories (mood disorders, substance-related disorders, etc.) in the *DSM–IV*

(American Psychiatric Association, 1994). The symptoms of some of the disorders are primarily physiological (e.g., breathing difficulties), others are characterized by avoidance (e.g., phobias), and others primarily consist of cognitive symptoms, such as worries and obsessions. A large number of efficacious treatments for anxiety disorders are in use, and a review of these is beyond the scope of this introduction. Although there are treatments that have been demonstrated to be efficacious for the anxiety disorders covered in this book (Social Anxiety Disorder, Panic Disorder [PD], and Generalized Anxiety Disorder [GAD]), few focus as much as CBASP on the consequences of the patient's behavior or the interpersonal difficulties that arise from the disorder.

CBASP emphasizes social problems and interpersonal relationships—realms of functioning specifically compromised in persons suffering from social anxiety. Chapter 9 demonstrates how CBASP can be easily incorporated—and in fact dovetails nicely—with existing empirically validated treatments for Social Anxiety Disorder (e.g., exposure). Moreover, the incremental efficacy of integrating the present approach is depicted in the transcripts of actual therapy sessions. CBASP effectively targets the specific behaviors and cognitions that contribute to long-term avoidance of social interactions, such that endured or thwarted anxiety is regularly attained across a variety of interpersonal contexts.

Little modification of the CBASP approach is actually needed to effectively target the maladaptive cognitions and behaviors that maintain both PD and GAD. Chapter 7 demonstrates that CBASP's emphasis on *specific* situations enhances CBASP's use as an in-session means to manage the often diffuse, unfocused anxiety symptoms associated with each of these conditions.

Parents, Children, and Couples

Parents of children with behavior disorders often focus on the need to change the child's behavior, without fully recognizing the role that their own thoughts and behaviors play in the perpetuation of family conflicts. Chapter 8 summarizes existing empirically validated treatments for externalizing behavior disorders, and the authors argue for the incorporation of CBASP into these treatments. The unmodified use of CBASP with parents in a group therapy setting is a demonstrated, effective means for positively changing parents' thoughts and behaviors, resulting in improvement not only in children's behaviors but also in overall family functioning.

1. COGNITIVE BEHAVIORAL ANALYSIS SYSTEM

Social skills deficits are common among children with a variety of behavioral problems, including Attention-Deficit/Hyperactivity Disorder, Oppositional Defiant Disorder, and Conduct Disorder. Children with these disorders often engage in negative behaviors that may be intended to gain attention but actually result in a lack of peer acceptance and, ultimately, peer rejection. Chapter 9 demonstrates how CBASP can be modified for use with children in both the individual and the group therapeutic setting. The modification of CBASP is described with particular emphasis on the analysis of the behavioral aspects of the treatment. Consideration of children's own thoughts and feelings as well as the thoughts and feelings of others is also stressed in the modification of the technique.

Treating couples in psychotherapy presents unique challenges, particularly because the couple is generally seeking treatment for relationship difficulties; however, these problems may be confounded by one—or both—partner's own psychopathology. Although there is not yet an official diagnosis assigned to couples who seek treatment (though there may be in future editions of the *DSM*), they are categorized as having a partner-relational problem, which is defined as a pattern of interaction between spouses or partners characterized by communication problems. Chapter 10 provides a review of the available treatment approaches for distressed couples. Although the principles of CBASP are consistent with already available treatments, this chapter demonstrates the unique use of the treatment, in which couple distress is the primary focus and individual distress is addressed indirectly.

Other Issues and Groups

Although it is not an independently diagnosable condition, excessive or uncontrolled anger constitutes a critical feature of many adult and childhood psychiatric disorders and can significantly interfere with several domains of life functioning. Chapter 11 explores the phenomenon of anger and briefly summarizes existing anger management techniques. The comparative use of CBASP is highlighted by its attention to the cognitive, emotional, and behavioral experience of anger, its straightforward integration of relaxation, and its inherently nonconfrontational approach, which makes it particularly amenable to clients prone to anger. The successful application of CBASP to anger management is illustrated in two case examples drawn from vastly different populations: an outpatient university clinic and a residential juvenile detention facility.

The use of CBASP is certainly not restricted to the outpatient clinic; rather, CBASP may be effectively applied within other settings, including correctional settings. Chapter 12 describes the interpersonal, emotional, and behavioral problems often encountered by prison inmates and forensic hospital inpatients and demonstrates, via session transcripts, how CBASP may be effectively applied to address the issues unique to incarcerated populations. A brief discussion of potential barriers to the implementation of mental health treatment in general, and CBASP in particular, within correctional settings is also provided.

The purpose of this book is to provide clinicians and other mental health care providers with a practical foundation for implementing CBASP with patients diagnosed with a variety of psychological difficulties and disorders. The modification and adaptation of CBASP is described in a straightforward fashion so that it can be easily used by those who lack formal training in its implementation. CBASP has been shown to be a time-limited, efficient treatment for patients diagnosed with depression; however, in this book, we demonstrate its potential with a variety of disorders.

PART I

Personality Disorders

Chapter 2

Schizotypal Personality Disorder*

Schizotypal Personality Disorder is identified by a pattern of maladaptive interpersonal behavior, characterized by specific cognitive and behavioral symptoms. Previous studies indicate this disorder can be successfully treated with Cognitive Behavioral Therapy. This chapter describes modifications of CBASP that increase the use of this technique to Schizotypal Personality Disorder. A case is presented that illustrates the application of specific components of this treatment (e.g., Situational Analysis) for reduction of these symptoms. A time-limited application of this treatment led to a significant reduction in symptom expression despite the long-standing nature of these symptoms in the patient.

Schizotypal Personality Disorder (STPD) is a pattern of maladaptive interpersonal behavior, characterized by certain cognitive (e.g., stereotyped thought, magical thinking) and behavioral (e.g., tangential/circumstantial speech, odd/eccentric) symptoms. These symptoms may result in extreme discomfort and a diminished capacity to form close relationships, beginning in early adulthood and evident across various situational contexts (American Psychiatric Association, 1994). Despite the seeming amenability of STPD symptoms to cognitive-behavioral intervention, this mode of treatment has been largely neglected. This apparent oversight may owe to the resemblance of STPD symptoms to Schizophrenia, a disorder generally accepted as biologically based and optimally treated with medication. Although other psychotherapy approaches have traditionally been applied, there is as yet no empirically validated treatment for STPD (Nathan &

---

*The primary authors contributing to this chapter were Maureen Lyons Reardon, Scharles C. Petty, and Thomas E. Joiner, Jr.

Gorman, 1998). However, the structure inherent in the Cognitive Behavioral Analysis System of Psychotherapy (CBASP; McCullough, 2000) makes it especially well suited to address STPD symptomatology.

HISTORY OF STPD TREATMENT

STPD has long been considered a Schizophrenia spectrum disorder (Benjamin, 1993), and providing some support for this view, the *Diagnostic and Statistical Manual of Mental Disorders–Fourth Edition* (*DSM–IV;* American Psychiatric Association, 1994) Cluster A personality disorders (i.e., STPD, schizoid, paranoid) are frequently present in the first-degree relatives of schizophrenics (Kendler, Masterson, Ungaro, & Davis, 1984). In view of this apparent relationship, it perhaps comes as little surprise that STPD has been successfully treated with low-dose neuroleptic antipsychotic medications. Though not effective for all STPD patients, several studies have shown that antipsychotic medications can be moderately effective in reducing STPD symptoms, such as ideas of reference, odd communication, social isolation, suspiciousness, and anxiety (Goldberg et al., 1986; Hymowitz, Frances, Jacobsberg, Sickles, & Hoyt, 1986; Schultz, Schultz, & Wilson, 1988).

Although psychodynamic approaches have also been traditionally applied, there exists little support for their clinical effectiveness with STPD (Siever & Kendler, 1986). Some clinicians believe that persons with STPD can benefit from dynamically oriented psychotherapy that focuses not on interpretation of conflict but on the internalization of a therapeutic relationship (Gabbard, 2000; Sperry, 1995). In other words, the therapist works to dissolve the rigid, internalized maladaptive attachment with early caregivers by providing an appropriate and corrective emotional experience in therapy. Others (Wainberg, Keefe, & Siever, 1995) contend that such exploratory psychotherapies are ineffective for STPD, arguing for more structured approaches (i.e., psychoeducation, reality testing, and interpersonal boundary reinforcement).

Based on Millon's (1981) view that STPD may be considered an extreme form of Schizoid Personality Disorder or Avoidant Personality Disorder, some have argued that the recommended interventions for these disorders also might be therapeutic for persons with STPD (e.g., Freeman, Pretzer, Fleming, & Simon, 1990). These approaches generally involve social skills training (e.g., role play) and graded exposure to social inter-

2. SCHIZOTYPAL PERSONALITY DISORDER 17

actions (Crits-Christoph, 1998), with the goal of encouraging a more positive view of social interactions through practice. Furthermore, the characteristic features of STPD, such as magical or illogical thinking, may require incorporating techniques successfully applied with schizophrenic patients. Some examples may include interventions aimed at enhancement of social skills, reduction of anxiety, and the improvement of problem-solving skills. Once improvement in behavior and thought oddities is achieved, these treatments for schizoid or avoidant personality disordered patients can then be effectively used in the treatment of STPD.

Interventions for STPD have been mainly behavioral in focus, with a primary emphasis on skills training rather than thought monitoring and development of appropriate responses to thoughts (Bellack & Hersen, 1985). The apparent emphasis on behavioral techniques is consistent with the notion that the bizarre thought processes associated with STPD may make purely cognitive techniques difficult and impractical (Freeman et al., 1990). Nonetheless, several recent randomized and controlled studies lend support for the use of cognitive therapy in the treatment of Schizophrenia (see Beck & Rector, 2000). The most successful therapies use a combination of cognitive and behavioral techniques to address distress associated with positive (e.g., hallucinations, delusions) or negative (e.g., flat affect, social withdrawal) symptoms, coping skills and symptom management, and the sense of alienation and stigma associated with mental illness (Haddock et al., 1998). Thus, it could be argued that if such interventions constitute efficacious treatment for a disorder as serious as Schizophrenia, similar techniques should be at least as effective in treating the relatively less severe but functionally similar symptoms associated with STPD.

In this vein, CBASP appears to be a particularly promising approach to the treatment of STPD symptoms. First, personality disordered patients repeatedly encounter situations that result in undesirable outcomes, and CBASP is designed to assist patients in identifying the thoughts and behaviors that are contributing to the unwanted outcomes in specific situations. Second, CBASP involves regular completion of the Coping Survey Questionnaire (CSQ), which aims, through detailed examination of stressful situations, to increase patients' control over life events to better manage their interpersonal environment. The CSQ summarizes the CBASP steps in simple form. Separate examination of behaviors and thoughts, connected to specific outcomes, can make complex and abstract life events simpler and more concrete; this method better accommodates the impaired thought processes (i.e., stereotypic, rigid) common to STPD pathology.

More important, the CBASP methods organize the therapy session, which helps to combat symptomatic tangential thought processes.

THERAPEUTIC STRUCTURE: APPLICATION OF A MODIFIED CBASP APPROACH FOR STPD

We recommend several modifications to the general CBASP approach to address the characteristic symptoms of STPD. First, STPD patients should be encouraged to select a particularly specific and brief slice of time for each CSQ. To evaluate adherence to this direction and correct any lapses thereof, patients can be asked to record the duration of selected situations (in minutes). Sentence limitations can also be imposed to reduce the number of loose associations generated for each item. Adopting a directive, sometimes interruptive, therapeutic style may help to focus the session and reduce irrelevant commentary. Second, because some STPD patients may be inclined to muddle the Desired Outcome (DO) with the description of the situation, they should be specifically directed not to do so. Such explicit instruction and separation may help to minimize STPD patients' confusion. Third, a restriction on the total number of cognitions can be imposed to effectively reduce tangential thought processes. Also, to emphasize that not all thoughts equally contribute to the perception of a situation, patients can be asked to rate each thought on a scale of 1 (*least applicable*) to 10 (*most applicable*). Fourth, the characteristically odd, eccentric behavior symptomatic of STPD often contributes significantly to STPD patients' ineffective navigation of social situations and should be afforded a prominent role in treatment. Additionally, queries concerning communication behavior in each situation can be separated into verbal and nonverbal behavior to make these queries especially concrete. We find it helpful to inquire specifically about nonverbal behaviors identified by Alberti and Emmons (1995) as critical to assertive communication (e.g., eye contact, body posture).

Additionally, therapists should consider the relative degree to which the STPD patient's behaviors and thoughts contribute to his or her maladaptive interpersonal style and accordingly afford greater initial focus to therapeutic interventions addressing the more severe domain of pathology (i.e., behaviors or thoughts). Setting a time limit for therapy may also help set boundaries for therapy, increase motivation for change, and encourage generalization of therapeutic gains outside the therapy setting. Such time limits may be helpful not only for STPD patients with long treatment histories but also for those in early treatment. Of course, time limits should not be rigidly enforced but revisited periodically to ensure sufficient progress has been made to justify termination.

Finally, STPD patients should be encouraged to seek feedback from others in terms of their impressions of communications after completion of a CSQ. In-session communications with the therapist may be used as material for CBASP, thereby permitting immediate feedback. This affords the opportunity to explore, in session, the effectiveness of patients' communications, and, if ineffective, how they could be improved. The use of the therapeutic relationship is considered particularly important in the treatment of STPD, helping the patient to foster genuine connections with others.

The following case description illustrates the therapeutic potential of applying these CBASP modifications in the treatment of STPD.

CASE EXAMPLE

Stan is a middle-aged, never-married, self-employed White man, who has lived alone for most of his adult life. He has a long history of mental illness dating back to his childhood, during which time he was reportedly subjected to unimaginable physical and sexual abuse by several close relatives. As a result, Stan has suffered from symptoms of Post-Traumatic Stress Disorder (PTSD), particularly nightmares, off and on for the past 20 years.

When Stan commenced the therapy described here, he held a strong conviction of inferiority. He insisted, "[I] am defective," a "smashed person," unworthy of most others' attention. These opinions appeared to hold, especially for those persons whom he perceived as attractive, educated, and "together." Stan commonly categorized people in this fashion, perhaps promoting a sense of separation and differentness from others. His social network was largely restricted to a few co-workers and a female friend for whom he reported only platonic interests. He further showed little recognition of the impact of his behaviors or statements on his associates. His approach to meeting women was rather haphazard and almost accidental, but he idealized these encounters as magical. This is certainly consistent with cognitions typical of STPD (e.g., "There are reasons for everything, things don't happen by chance" [Beck & Freeman,

1990, p. 140]). Moreover, his description of his relationships was noticeably absent any depth or intimacy. Persons whom Stan identified as friends were typically more characteristic of acquaintances or casual contacts, suggesting a rather superficial understanding of what constituted closeness with others.

Stan also exhibited noticeably odd behaviors that compromised his communications with others, characteristics quite typical of STPD pathology. For example, Stan tended to vocalize every thought that occurred to him when explaining a situation, as if each were equally important to the communication. He showed particular difficulty staying focused and generally responded to questions in a rambling, tangential manner. His speech had the quality of a radio announcer, and, in fact, Stan later admitted that he had attempted to model a local disc jockey's pattern of speech. Stan also referred to himself pluralistically, as "we" or "ourselves," and described ostensible feelings of social discomfort as being "out of [my] body." Stan offered little eye contact and initially sat himself in a position perpendicular to the therapist.

Due to poor documentation and communication between various treatment providers, the details of Stan's extensive encounters with the mental health system are sketchy at best. A review of his file indicates he first entered treatment in 1979, at which time symptoms of depressed mood, frequent crying spells, low self-image, sleep disturbance (insomnia), impaired concentration, suicidal ideation, and parental conflict dominated his clinical presentation. Over the next 3 years, Stan participated in both individual and group therapy and was prescribed Amitriptyline (an antidepressant) and Midrin (for migraines). During this time, Stan's symptoms of depression improved, and he finished junior college and was accepted to a major state university. Stan immediately sought treatment on arrival at the university and was seen by several therapists in the community. A predominantly psychoanalytic approach had been used to combat his recurrent depression and anxiety symptoms as well as to improve his socialization.

Stan was first seen by our training clinic in 1985. Although the precise targets of intervention were inadequately reflected in his chart, the approaches to treatment over the next 3 years were identified as cognitive restructuring, systematic desensitization, relaxation training, stress management, and social skills training. In 1988, Stan was diagnosed with Multiple Personality Disorder (i.e., Dissociative Identity Disorder), and an age-regression approach was used to work through his suppressed traumatic childhood. Over the 13 years Stan received treatment, he was transferred 12 times due to his therapists' completion of their graduate clinical training requirements. By 1991, the approach to his symptoms was again identified as cognitive-behavioral with a relaxation-training component.

Stan was not diagnosed with STPD until 1994. Over the next several years, Stan was treated by four therapists who focused on encouraging him to openly express emotions and to gain insight into his impact on others. Although apparently helpful in combating his depression and overt anxiety symptoms, none of these therapies adequately addressed the features of STPD that compromised his social functioning. Indeed, a prolonged reliance on therapy as the primary forum for emotional expression and social interaction may have served to further isolate him from social contacts outside the therapy setting.

Course of Treatment: Symptoms and Outcomes

A 6-month time-limited, modified CBASP approach was selected to address the apparent shortcomings of his previous therapies. We first targeted Stan's unusual nonverbal presentation and its impact on his communication skills. As an adjunct bibliotherapy, Stan was encouraged to read pertinent sections of *Your Perfect Right* (Alberti & Emmons, 1995), which describes the role of nonverbal behavior in communication. As he achieved substantial progress in behavioral domains (i.e., communication skills), we increasingly emphasized the role of his maladaptive cognitions in his limited social interactions outside the therapy setting. This was considered particularly important to his transition from a long-term reliance on therapy as the primary avenue of social expression to more appropriate, outside interpersonal contacts. Finally, issues pertinent to his termination were actively addressed in session, not only to firm up boundaries and increase motivation for change but also to offer him a chance to practice expression of emotions with the therapist. The therapeutic relationship holds the potential to model appropriate social interaction and also can help foster interpersonal connectedness.

It should be noted that although we present Stan's therapy in terms of these three targets of intervention, they should not be considered separate phases of treatment. That is, despite gradual shifts in the emphasis of CBASP intervention, as progress in each domain became evident, his odd behaviors, maladaptive cognitions, and termination issues were addressed throughout his therapy.

EMPHASIS: COMMUNICATION SKILLS

As stated previously, Stan initially sat himself in a position sideways relative to the therapist. Stan readily provided a rationale for this behavior by stating, "I guess I'm used to my house . . . I always sit on the right side, I'm left-handed. I guess I do just about everything that way." He further indicated that he needed to have a desk and used the windowsill on the opposite side of the therapy room for this purpose. This behavior persisted in the next session, despite the therapist's experiment in which a therapy room without windows was selected. In addition, Stan rarely offered regular eye contact when speaking with others, including the therapist. Rather than the therapist adjusting to Stan's maladaptive behaviors, these behaviors were regularly addressed in the context of CBASP using Stan's DO of communicating effectively with the therapist. Regular feedback concerning the effectiveness of his interactions was provided. These efforts were met with some resistance at first, and Stan arrived a few minutes late for the next several sessions. During his fifth session, the following dialogue occurred:

Therapist: For example . . . if you take you and me. I would find it easier for us to relate and for me to relate to other people when they're facing me, looking at me, and engaged with me. That's why I brought up the chair thing.

Stan: Yeah I had others ask about that, or they say "you don't look that much," and it's hard to . . .

Therapist: (*interrupting*) What do you think that means?

Stan: When they ask or what does it mean for me? (*some cognitive dysregulation here*)

Therapist: What it means for you.

Stan: What do I think it means to me or what do I think it means for them?

2. SCHIZOTYPAL PERSONALITY DISORDER

Therapist: (*make specific*) Why don't we take it when they say it. How does that make you feel then?

Stan: I would say that . . . that would make you feel in control and maybe superior in a way. More skilled, aware of social things, and . . .

Therapist: Well, how does it? I mean, I can see what you see it can do for you. But . . .

Stan: No. That's what it means for you.

Therapist: What do you mean? I'm not following. (*clarification if thought processes are unclear*)

Stan: I always have thought of a counselor (*i.e., therapist*) as real socially skilled, polished, in control of themselves . . .

Therapist: So what does it mean when people tell you that you're not doing those things?

Stan: I guess that I have a lot more to learn about myself and that I still have good little habits to overcome. Just a lot of work to do.

Therapist: (*therapy relationship as model*) Right now you're looking at me. We're talking. When you're looking at me, what's going on . . . how do you feel? Is it uncomfortable?

Stan: Uncomfortable, maybe. (*pause*) Challenging I guess.

Therapist: Because you're really trying?

Stan: Trying to. It's real hard to get myself to feel together and organized, engaged with someone, to feel equal. That's the hardest part, just feeling equal.

Therapist: You feel someone has the upper edge on you in some way?

Stan: I've got that, no doubt about that.

Therapist: What would it take for you to start to do those things, like orienting yourself to other people, looking at them when they talk to you—what would it take?

Stan: Wow. (*pause*) I guess reading more about it, practicing it.

Therapist: Practice. Yeah, that's the big one. Sounds like you know what it could do for you.

Stan: Yeah, that's not easy stuff to do, but . . .

Therapist: I'm not saying that.

Stan: Not much time to get all that stuff together.

Therapist: What do you mean "not that much time"?

Stan: Well, time with us is running out. Time goes so fast. Stuff with the book, that's the kind of stuff—and my little assignments here. You don't want to just say, "Oh, I'll do it later." That means do it now as best you can. And I got to make time. That's hard to sit down with (*Ms. X*) and say this may sound really weird, but let

> me go over this list of stuff to talk about. (*chuckles*) I'll just have
> to make time to do it and present it to somebody. And (*grabbing
> his completed CSQ*) I found someone I could do it with.

The preceding exchange not only illustrates how Stan's core cognitions of inferiority are closely linked to his oddities of behavior but also supports our contention that our imposition of a time limit helped to motivate change. In the following session, Stan arrived promptly and stated, "I was thinking about what you said, and so this week . . ." He proceeded to pick up a chair from the opposite side of the room and sat himself face to face with the therapist for the first time. This behavior change persisted throughout the remainder of his therapy.

By his 10th session, it became clear that these CBASP interventions had resulted in significant improvement: Stan evidenced an increased awareness of the connection between his behaviors, thoughts, and consequent outcomes. During this session, Stan presented a CSQ in which he was able to achieve his DO regarding a renewal of a previous friendship with a male friend. In discussing his nonverbal communication in the situation, he acknowledged that he noticed his eye contact was fleeting at times. Importantly, however, he stated that he paid particular attention to his presentation because, he stated, "the better [my] eye contact, the more honest and sincere [I] can be with him."

In addition, the structure imposed on the therapy sessions appeared to improve Stan's ability to stay focused on the content of the session, and his tangential communications were greatly reduced. Indeed, Stan was increasingly able to identify when a particular thought was not important to his communications and stop himself from pursuing inappropriate, unhelpful lines of discussion. At one point, in Session 14, for example, Stan caught himself without therapist direct intervention, "Yes, well. We can talk about that later. The important thing is . . ." In-session improvements in nonverbal communication gradually generalized to social interactions outside of therapy, as he increasingly began to achieve his DOs related to taking appropriate social risks. He consistently completed CSQ homework that illustrated the successful initiation of appropriate conversations with others and was better able to follow the conventions of social interaction. Accordingly, the focus of therapy shifted to addressing the maladaptive cognitions that impeded his progress in this domain,

2. SCHIZOTYPAL PERSONALITY DISORDER

while continuing to monitor his behavioral gains in the context of CBASP.

EMPHASIS: COGNITIONS

To some extent, the improvements in Stan's behavioral presentation generalized to his maladaptive cognitions, providing him with a new sense of self-efficacy for effectively engaging in social situations. Earlier in treatment, Stan related such core thought processes as "I feel way too self-conscious," "I don't belong here," "This [social interaction] isn't easy for me," and "I can't confront someone if he's angry with me." These cognitions were simply addressed in the context of CBASP as unhelpful in attaining his reported DOs to communicate effectively in various specific situations. Continued practice and rehearsal of these cognitions in specific social interactions, along with more frequent achievement of his DOs, resulted in significant improvement in Stan's previously "smashed" self-image. Over the course of his therapy, Stan generated a list of positive thoughts that facilitated effective social interactions outside of the therapy setting (see Table 2.1).

TABLE 2.1
Summary of Revised Cognitions of Self-Image and Self-Efficacy

Self-Image	Self-Efficacy
"Other people report that I am normal."	"It's not hard to communicate well."
"I'm desired and valued from people."	"I'm not always focused, but I am learning and improving my ability to be focused and orderly."
"I treat people with respect."	
"I'm knowledgeable and generous."	"I've learned to pay attention to what (my) self is telling (my)self and not to just do nothing."
"I am a good listener."	
	"I'm going to be myself, be the best me that I can be, and will try to be aware, as much as possible, of other people involved."
	"I've improved a lot over the years; I've fought for it, fought hard and will continue to fight."
	"Whatever his attitude is, good or bad, I can handle it."

As an example of this progress, while reviewing his CSQ assignment during his 14th session, Stan generated several alternate interpretations that clearly would have helped him achieve his DO in an interaction with several women during a business-related exposition where he presented his work. The therapist jotted down his thoughts and repeatedly tied them to his DO to demonstrate a good social interaction:

Therapist: Well, okay, so you got a couple of thoughts here that sound a whole lot better than the ones on the previous page (*the original CSQ homework*) that you might just want to consider changing to, or at least trying to think of, when you are about to approach someone and meet with them. They are (*reviewing notes*): "Others report that I am normal" and "I am desired and valued from people."

Stan: Yeah. And they said that I had obviously studied that stuff for years—which I had, like 30 years already—and that they were glad that I take time to go see them. Because there's one guy there that I know very well that's a brilliant man but also a very arrogant man. [They said] they felt really put off by him, intimidated, and not at all able to be themselves.

Therapist: Hmm . . . That . . . that doesn't seem to fit with your last one here, and that's probably why you got the 50% one here. (*rating of degree of thought applicability to the situation*)

Stan: Which one was that?

Therapist: (*reading*) "I am an extremely self-centered person."

Stan: Well, there's a good example of how you can turn exactly that into something positive. Which is a fine line, because I have been real self-centered and a lot of it is from learning all that stuff and kind of doing my own PhD with learning information, writing it, and sharing it. There's been a lot of being self-centered, but if you take time for someone . . .

Therapist: (*interrupting*) Sounds like to me what they were saying is "you're a pretty knowledgeable person in this area, seems like you've studied a lot, and you took the time to come out and help us."

Stan: That's the key.

Therapist: Well, what would you say about somebody who's knowledgeable and willing to take the time to help other people?

Stan: You treat them with respect . . . don't talk down at them. Make them feel like any counselor would, like they're the most important person right then.

Therapist: (*writing*) "I treat people with respect."

2. SCHIZOTYPAL PERSONALITY DISORDER

Stan: And "importance," too.

Therapist: "I treat people with respect and importance." Does that thought help you get what you want, which is to have a good interaction with people?

Stan: That's what I got from them, yeah.

By his 18th session, Stan had furnished a completed CSQ in which he described a conversation with a waitress at a local restaurant. He noted his DO as "I wanted to have a casual but friendly conversation with her." Particularly noteworthy, arguably all of his interpretations in this situation served to help him achieve this desired end—for example, "she doesn't mind my being here," "she's more approachable," "it's okay for me to sit down with her," and "I'm feeling together, real together," "I'm prepared." His nonverbal behaviors were also consistently likely to help him get what he wanted in this situation. Importantly, Stan perceived this interaction as successful, and feedback that he subsequently solicited from the waitress supported this interpretation.

Despite his apparent improvements in behaviors and cognitions, however, Stan continued to categorize people in terms of their perceived value in relation to himself, contending that most others were unapproachable. These interpretations may have caused Stan to avoid social interactions with those persons he perceived as somehow more valuable than him. In the context of CBASP, these thoughts can simply be considered a contributing factor in his failure to achieve his DOs of social interaction. Although these cognitions were addressed repeatedly in the context of his CSQ assignments, it was not until his 22nd session that Stan reported a particularly enlightening experience. He told the therapist that he had recently seen a speed trap, and no sooner did he say to himself, "Boy, am [I] glad [I'm] not one of those people who gets pulled over" that he "saw blue lights in [his] rearview mirror." Stan reported that he subsequently began maintaining a log of how many times he made negative attributions about people in an effort to differentiate himself from them, observing that he did so at least 10 times per day. He further estimated that he had made "about 14,000 negative attributions in 40 years." Stan commented that replacing such thoughts with positive attributions would be a slow process and would "not be a magical change." In connection with the cognitions characteristic of STPD, in which such experiences are likely to be viewed as having magical implications (Beck & Freeman, 1990), Stan's practical and realistic view of this change process was considered to mark significant progress. Ultimately, Stan concluded that he would use his "speedometer to remind [him] of how [he is] like other people." This demonstrates Stan's increasing reliance on himself, as opposed to therapy, as the resource for altering his maladaptive cognitions.

EMPHASIS: TERMINATION

When the issue of termination was readdressed in Session 18, Stan responded in a manner consistent with the intended goal of this time-limited therapeutic approach, "It's time to narrow down to work that would be risky." Although time-limited, structured therapy motivates substantial change in a short period of time, some regressions are to be expected. For example, Stan arrived early for his 23rd session, using his time in the waiting room to organize his thoughts. He initially turned his chair away from the therapist but then rearranged his chair stating, "[I'm] not doing this right. We worked on this in the beginning. [I'm] not communicating." Although he was speaking coherently from the therapist's standpoint, he repeatedly stated that he was not. His approach to this session did not appear to be reflective of a defensive effort to avoid termination but rather of an active, albeit somewhat rigid, effort to make himself feel less scattered. Such awareness and effort could be viewed as progress, demonstrating his increased reliance on himself, rather than the therapist, to improve his focus and communication. Indeed, some discomfort can be expected, considering the significant adjustments he had made in his life.

The emotions surrounding his termination as well as personal loss of therapist were addressed in session using CBASP. Such an approach affords the therapist the opportunity to explore, in session, the effectiveness of Stan's communications and, if ineffective, provide immediate feedback on how the communication could be improved. In addition, by making the loss of his therapist personal, the therapist hoped to unconstrict Stan's affect and provide him with a sense of in-the-moment interpersonal connectedness. Not surprisingly, Stan initially struggled to communicate negative emotions concerning this loss. He often avoided discussion of losing the therapist by referring to her as just one of many therapists or referring to the clinic in general. In keeping with the general approach to his therapy, Stan was redirected. Perhaps due to his prior routine transfers in therapy, he struggled to understand the concept and value of active termination and of saying good-bye.

Also, perhaps not unexpected, Stan cancelled his last session by leaving a message to inform the therapist of his thanks and well-being. With some persuasion, however, he agreed to come in for a final session. Emphasis was placed on the importance of saying good-bye, despite its built-in complication of emotions, and the therapist highlighted how a phone message would make such important communications impossible. During his termination session, Stan's affect was less restricted. He asked appropriate questions with minimal digressions and demonstrated excellent eye contact and appropriate nonverbal behavior. At the session's conclusion, the therapist offered Stan a handshake, to which Stan looked directly at the therapist (i.e., good eye contact), with some tearfulness, the first emotions surrounding termination yet expressed, he gestured for a hug. From a professional standpoint, this provided a mark of substantial progress for this patient in terms of his capacity for personal connection.

Stan was able to achieve significant progress in his nonverbal social presentation, as evidenced by his improved eye contact and permanent behavioral adjustment in seating position. His communication skills were vastly enhanced by improvements in his thought processes (e.g., tangentiality, loose associations). Most important, after just 24 sessions of CBASP, Stan was able to make a successful transition out of therapy, which to this point had served as his primary outlet for social interaction for much of his adult life.

POTENTIAL OBSTACLES TO CBASP APPLICATIONS TO STPD

Although the proposed changes to CBASP are likely to greatly improve the focus and structure of sessions with the STPD patient, successful implementation of this approach may require some adjustment to one's typical therapeutic style. As in the present case, a directive, sometimes interruptive, style must be adopted early in treatment to reduce symptomatic tangential thoughts. Such efforts may seem awkward and at times uncomfortable for therapists not accustomed to communicating with their patients in this manner. It is imperative that therapists adopting this approach carefully balance directive efforts to focus sessions against the critical efforts to provide the patient with an in-session model of communication. In other words, therapists must be careful not to suggest that interruption of others is socially appropriate. Instead, the therapist's directive disruption of the patient's loose associations should be conducted only with mindful intention of educating the patient about what is essential to the description of a particular situation. CBASP is helpful in delineating this subtle distinction, making it immediately clear how tangential thoughts or certain social behaviors may be only remotely related, or at times completely unrelated, to the DOs and thus not helpful in the context of most social communications.

As symptoms improve, a less directive and interruptive style may be needed to focus the therapy session. Over time, the patient should be encouraged to take more of the lead in session. Initially, for example, the therapist read and reviewed Stan's assignments in session. Later, Stan was asked to review the assignment as the therapist took notes. This transaction was then explored as in-session communication, subject to CBASP and feedback from the therapist regarding the effectiveness of Stan's communication. To effectively use the therapeutic relationship in this context, genuineness on the part of the therapist is needed to make the relationship both important and real—a challenge for STPD patients, who may not readily view any persons in this manner.

Additionally, becoming acquainted with the odd manner in which STPD patients communicate their thoughts and behaviors may pose an additional challenge for the inexperienced therapist, particularly early in treatment when idiosyncrasies of behavior can seem quite foreign. To ensure proper understanding, the therapist should attempt to summarize the patient's cognitions using more common wording. The therapist may also wish to consider offering feedback on these translations of the patient's self-reported cognitions, particularly if they are thought to impede effective communication.

Another issue that may emerge in the treatment of STPD is the use of psychiatric medications. As noted previously, many atypical neuroleptic medications appear to be effective for some of the pseudoschizophrenia symptoms of STPD. Thus, along with a psychiatrist and the STPD patient, therapists should afford psychiatric medications due consideration as a viable adjunct treatment. In the present case, Stan stopped

2. SCHIZOTYPAL PERSONALITY DISORDER

taking his prescriptions for Risperdal (antipsychotic) and Imipramine (antidepressant) in the months prior to the start of current treatment. Accordingly, medication compliance was encouraged as an adjunct to his therapy, helping him to clear his thoughts. By Session 4, Stan had begun taking Risperdal again and reported improvements in sleep and fewer nightmares and intrusive thoughts of his past abuse history (however, we believe it would be an inferential mistake to attribute Stan's success to his medications because medications taken before CBASP had not resulted in much improvement).

In fact, few patients present with STPD symptoms in isolation; mood, anxiety, and other personality symptoms commonly cooccur with this condition. In the present case, Stan's PTSD remained in partial remission throughout much of his treatment. Like many disorders with this clinical status, occasional relapses of symptoms can and did occur. Whenever possible, CBASP was used at these times, particularly if the symptoms were situation specific and thus readily amenable to this approach. This is the preferred approach to addressing comorbid pathology because, as noted elsewhere in this text, CBASP is quite flexible for many psychological conditions and everyday problems. Other times, however, a more general cognitive-behavioral intervention was employed with Stan to address these symptoms. A description of these interventions is clearly beyond the scope of the present discussion, but the interested reader is referred to Resick and Calhoun (2001) for information on an effective treatment for PTSD.

Given that STPD patients may not be aware of the impact of their odd behaviors on their life situation, it is likely that their perception of progress in this regard may vary widely from that of the therapist. For example, during Stan's 10th session, he was asked to rate his progress in his nonverbal behaviors on a scale of 1 = *I need work* to 4 = *okay* to 7 = *excellent.* In contrast with observations of his improvement by his therapist and supervisor, Stan rated all but gestures as in need of some work (range 2.5–3.5). This discrepancy was thought to reflect Stan's maladaptive self-cognitions, which had, by this point, only recently constituted the emphasis of CBASP intervention. As can be seen in Table 2.1, however, with repeated practice and more frequent achievement of his social DOs, Stan's self-efficacy had apparently caught up to his behaviors by the conclusion of his therapy. In this connection, it should be reiterated that therapists should make note of changes in observable behaviors and provide regular, in-session feedback concerning communication improvements. Of course, the process of CBASP yields successful interpersonal outcomes outside of therapy that even the least insightful cannot deny as progress.

The preceding case description clearly illustrates how the imposition of a directive, time-limited, structured CBASP protocol need not be impersonal and mechanical but quite therapeutic for persons with STPD. Although STPD patients may not be aware of their odd nonverbal social presentation, CBASP can enable their substantial progress in this regard (e.g., increasing eye contact). Moreover, improvements in thought processing (i.e., loosening of associations) are also made possible by the structure inherent in the CBASP method. Ultimately, the collaborative examination of interpretations in the context of CBASP serves to encourage the generalization of social experiences outside the therapy session. Although CBASP clearly awaits formal empirical evaluation as an STPD treatment, it appears to be a quite promising approach for persons with STPD, regardless of the duration or severity of personality dysfunction.

Chapter 3

Borderline Personality Disorder*

Borderline Personality Disorder has traditionally been considered among the more difficult disorders to treat, in part due to the interpersonal deficits patients with the disorder exhibit. This chapter summarizes the application of the Cognitive Behavioral Analysis System of Psychotherapy to Borderline Personality Disorder and suggests ways in which the approach complements existing treatments for Borderline Personality Disorder. The use of Situational Analysis is presented as a means of identifying and correcting maladaptive patterns of thinking and behaving that typify this disorder. A case example illustrates the implementation of this treatment and associated symptom reduction.

Borderline Personality Disorder (BPD) has been part of psychiatric nosology since the 1930s (Green, 1977). The *Diagnostic and Statistical Manual of Mental Disorders–Fourth Edition* (*DSM–IV;* American Psychiatric Association, 1994) conceptualizes BPD as an eclectic set of observed signs and reported characteristics that are derived from clinical reports and, to a lesser extent, from empirical research. In the *DSM–IV,* BPD is defined as "a pervasive pattern of instability of interpersonal relationships, self-image, and affects, and a marked impulsivity beginning by early adulthood and present in a variety of contexts" (p. 654). The patient must satisfy five (or more) of nine possible criteria to receive a diagnosis of BPD. The prevalence of BPD is approximately 2% in the general population and may be up to 30% to 60% in clinical populations with personality disorders (American Psychiatric Association, 1994). In addition, 75% of patients diagnosed

---

*The primary authors contributing to this chapter were Sarah A. Shultz and Keith F. Donohue.

with BPD are female (American Psychiatric Association, 1994). Although the *DSM–IV* approach has improved the diagnostic reliability considerably, the validity of the approach and its use in identifying patients with BPD has not gone unquestioned. Linehan (1993a) has advanced her own conceptualization of BPD based on a biosocial theory of the disorder. This conceptualization stresses the importance of the interaction between biological and social learning influences on the etiology and development of BPD.

Linehan's (1993a) conceptualization uses the *DSM–IV* criteria but organizes the symptoms into a set of dysregulated behavioral patterns that arise within five basic systems. Emotion or affective dysregulation refers to affective instability due to a marked reactivity of mood and inappropriate, intense, anger or difficulty controlling anger. Patients with BPD are likely to experience highly reactive emotional responses, with periods of depression, anxiety, and irritability, as well as intense anger. Behavioral dysregulation refers to impulsivity, including suicidal behavior and self-mutilating behavior. More specifically, impulsivity may include excessive spending, shoplifting, promiscuous sex, substance abuse, reckless driving, or binge eating. That patients with BPD are more likely than patients without the diagnosis to injure, mutilate, or kill themselves highlights the often extreme nature of impulsivity among those with BPD. Interpersonal dysregulation refers to a pattern of unstable and intense relationships and frantic efforts to avoid real or imagined abandonment. Patients with BPD are likely to be involved in chaotic relationships, find it extremely hard to let go of relationships, and often go to extreme lengths to avoid perceived abandonment. Self-dysregulation includes identity disturbance and chronic feelings of emptiness. Patients with BPD often report having no sense of self, feeling empty, or not knowing who they are. Finally, cognitive dysregulation includes paranoid ideation or dissociative symptoms, usually related to stress. Under stress, it is not uncommon for patients with this disorder to experience mild psychotic forms of thought disturbance, including depersonalization, dissociations, and delusions; however, these symptoms are generally transient and less severe when compared to symptoms of frank psychotic disorders (Linehan, 1993a).

TREATMENT OF BORDERLINE PERSONALITY DISORDER

Therapists have employed a variety of treatment approaches when confronted with the varied and often severe features of BPD. Central to early identification and conceptualization of the disorder, psychoanalytic approaches to the treatment of BPD have enjoyed an extensive history of application (for a review, see Linehan & Kehrer, 1993). Psychoanalytic approaches generally seek to expose and resolve latent psychic processes and help patients to better tolerate and manage their emotionality. Within session, the therapist observes and comments on the emotional tone of his or her interactions with the patient and offers interpretations of the latent processes that may underlie these emotions (Masterson & Klein, 1989). The patient must confront these interpretations and either agree or revise them with the therapist. This process allows patients to gain insight into the source of the strong emotional reactions that they experience and to develop mechanisms for tolerating and coping with these reactions.

Despite extensive clinical writing, relatively little research has been done to support the efficacy of psychodynamic approaches to treatment for BPD (Linehan & Kehrer, 1993). Many of these techniques were developed prior to the establishment of *DSM* criteria for BPD and are based on a psychoanalytic model of the disorder that includes a broader range of features than those included in the *DSM*. As a result, the sample of patients treated with psychodynamic approaches may be considered particularly heterogeneous and difficult to specify for research. In addition, psychodynamic approaches to treatment are designed to take place over several years of treatment, a span of time that most patients fail to complete. These factors help to explain why, despite the considerable influences that they have had on theory of BPD, psychodynamic approaches to treatment of this disorder have not been rigorously examined by empirical research.

Interpersonal approaches to treatment of BPD emphasize the interpersonal contexts in which the central features of BPD occur (Benjamin, 1993). These contexts include a history of traumatic abandonment, a chaotic lifestyle that involves repeated crises, experiences of attempts to exert autonomy that were met with attacks, and the assumption of a sick role that elicited nurturance. Benjamin's (1993) Structural Analysis of Social Behavior treats BPD by helping the patient to better understand and manage the patterns of interpersonal interaction in his or her life. Over the course of treatment, the therapist helps the patient to gain insight into these patterns of interaction and encourages the patient to give up those that lead to destructive outcomes. During this process, the therapist must be sensitive to the patient's fear of changing and to his or her sense of loss when giving up old patterns of interaction. Although interpersonal approaches have influenced the conceptualization and treatment of BPD, they are relatively new and have not been examined by empirical research.

Developed initially by Beck (Beck, Rush, Shaw, & Emery, 1987; Young, Beck, & Weinberger, 1993) as a treatment for depression, cognitive therapy has been applied to the treatment of personality disorders, including BPD (Beck & Freeman, 1990). The cognitive conceptualization of BPD includes both the negative cognitions that patients with BPD hold about themselves and their interpersonal relationships and the distorted processes of thinking in which they engage when evaluating situations. Together, these two broad features are thought to underlie and maintain the maladaptive patterns of emotional reactions and behavior that characterize BPD. Patients with BPD are thought to have negative cognitions that include the belief that the world is essentially dangerous and malevolent, that the patient is powerless and vulnerable to harm, and that the patient is inherently unacceptable or unlovable to others.

Perhaps the most significant cognitive distortion from this perspective is dichotomous thinking, in which the patient tends to interpret experiences in terms of extreme, mutually exclusive categories. For example, the patient may interpret an interpersonal encounter as either an unqualified success or an unmitigated failure. Because dichotomous thinking underlies many of the BPD patient's difficulties and serves to maintain his or her negative cognitions, the central focus of cognitive therapy for BPD is the reduction or elimination of this distorted process of thinking. The tendency to engage in dichotomous thinking (the very target of treatment) may lead BPD patients to alternately view the therapist as a supportive ally and as an unsupportive enemy. To overcome this difficulty, the therapist must first acknowledge the patient's difficulty in trusting him or her and then engage in a pattern of consistently trustworthy behavior. That is, the therapist must take extra care to be responsive to the patient and must respond consistently and patiently to his or her concerns. Once a trusting relationship is developed, the therapist must balance the need to respond to the patient's acute concerns (and thereby maintain the patient's trust in the therapist's responsiveness) and the need to focus on the long-term goals of therapy. Beck and Freeman (1990) suggested that cognitive therapy for BPD patients may be effective over the course of 1 to 2 years in decreasing dichotomous thinking and the negative cognitions that characterize BPD. Although they offer case examples of successful treatment, this approach to therapy has not yet been rigorously evaluated by empirical research.

Young, Beck, and Weinberger (1993) have expanded the basic principles of cognitive therapy to develop schema-focused therapy, which proposes that the cognitions that characterize personality disorders are elements of more broad and stable patterns of thinking that arise from early life experiences and expand over the course of development. Nine of these early maladaptive schemas that characterize BPD include abandonment/loss ("no one will care for me"), unlovability ("if people really knew me, they would not love me"), dependence ("I need someone to take care of me"), subjugation ("if I express how I feel, people will abandon or attack me"), mistrust ("people will hurt me, if I let them"), inadequate self-discipline ("I am unable to control myself"), fear of losing emotional control ("if I lose control of my emotions, something terrible will happen to me"), guilt ("I am a bad person"), and emotional deprivation ("no one is ever there for me"). Schema-focused therapy proceeds in a similar fashion to other forms of cognitive approaches to treatment. However, the therapist is directed to explore the operation of the characteristic BPD schemas behind the surface-level cognitions. The therapist then identifies these schemas for the patient and encourages the patient to challenge and revise them. Although it expands on the traditional model of cognitive therapy, schema-focused therapy has not yet been rigorously evaluated by empirical research.

Dialectical Behavioral Therapy (DBT) grew out of the application of cognitive-behavioral approaches to the treatment of BPD, particularly those patients with BPD who engage in chronic suicidal behavior (Linehan, 1993a; Linehan & Kehrer, 1993). Although both therapies address the influence that cognitions have on emotional processes, DBT adds additional emphasis on correcting the core dysfunction in emotional regulation that is thought to underlie BPD. According to a diathesis-stress model, due to an underlying diathesis making them vulnerable to strong emotional responses and stressors from interpersonal environments that invalidate their feelings, patients with BPD are prone to extreme patterns of emotional responding. DBT uses the construct of the dialectic (i.e., the balance between opposites) to organize treatment. At its most general level, DBT balances radical acceptance of the patient's condition against the need to seek change. To help the patient achieve this balance, the patient and the therapist engage in other, more specific dialectical processes, such as balancing validation of the patient's feelings against a pragmatic approach to problem solving and balancing reciprocal communication against irreverent communication between therapist and patient.

DBT is divided into the following components: individual sessions between patient and therapist, skills training groups for the patient, and telephone consultations between therapist and patient during crises. (Linehan, 1993a, suggests a group consultation for the therapist as a fourth component.) Individual sessions between patient and therapist involve explicit teaching of skills related to emotion regulation and implicit training in the form of chain analysis of events. In this latter element, the therapist and patient dismantle a distressing event that resulted in self-harming behavior. Chain analysis is designed to help detect points of intervention that can be used to avert self-harming behavior. This serves to validate the patient's experience, while also demonstrating the connection between thoughts and actions that lead to self-harming behavior. In this way, chain analysis reflects the overall dialectical balance between accepting the patient as he or she is and enabling change. Group sessions for the patient are designed to consolidate the gains made in individual sessions by relating them to skill modules for core mindfulness, emotion regulation, distress tolerance, and interpersonal effectiveness (Linehan, 1993b). In addition, patients are encouraged to contact the therapist during crises that occur between sessions to gain support and encouragement for the use of the skills taught in session.

DBT is an intensive approach to the treatment of severely disordered patients. Although its overall effectiveness and the relative contributions of its elements to treatment have been questioned (Scheel, 2000; Turner, 2000), it is the most rigorously evaluated treatment for BPD. Treatment studies indicate that BPD is effective in reducing some of the features associated with this disorder, particularly self-harming behavior (Westen, 2000).

Although it is not yet a well-established treatment, at this time the most empirically validated treatment for BPD is DBT. However, there are several aspects of DBT that make it difficult to conduct outside of a clinic designed for the implementation of DBT. For example, one of the essential components of DBT is skills training. It is recommended that skills training be conducted in a group format to reserve time in individual therapy for crisis intervention and attention to other issues (Linehan, 1993a). This is often difficult in small clinics, private practice environments, and in hospital settings. In addition, many of the concepts of DBT may be difficult to learn and incorporate into treatment, especially for beginning therapists.

APPLICATION OF CBASP TO BORDERLINE PERSONALITY DISORDER

In reviewing the literature on treatments for BPD, it is clear that the clinician has many options but no clearly preferred choice. Given this situation,

3. BORDERLINE PERSONALITY DISORDER

our attempts to advance another approach to treatment may seem questionable. However, our clinical work suggests that a treatment based on elements of the Cognitive Behavioral Analysis System of Psychotherapy (CBASP; McCullough, 2000) may hold significant advantages for working with patients with BPD. These patients often represent a challenge for therapists, one that is compounded by the challenge of mastering complex therapeutic models and applying them across often turbulent and inconsistent sessions that are typical of treatment. The CBASP approach to treatment offers a degree of simplicity while also incorporating many of the elements found in other forms of treatment.

The major therapeutic tool in CBASP is Situational Analysis (SA), a process that is recorded by the patient on the Coping Survey Questionnaire (CSQ) and then reviewed by the therapist in session (McCullough, 2000). Similar to the interpersonal model, CBASP is based on the assumption that the defining feature of BPD is a persistent pattern of unsuccessful interpersonal interactions. The main tool for correcting this pattern is the CSQ technique for SA, which is used in three distinct ways. First, the CSQ can be used to identify and modify maladaptive cognitions. The patient completes the CSQ for homework, which is then reviewed within session. Second, the CSQ can be used for crisis intervention between sessions. Finally, the CSQ can be used to understand and modify conflicts occurring between the therapist and the patient within session.

In the first case, special emphasis is placed on elements that have been gleaned from cognitive approaches to treatment. Our clinical work suggests that patients with BPD tend to evaluate Desired Outcomes (DOs) and Actual Outcomes (AOs) for interpersonal situations in ways that reflect the dichotomous thinking proposed by the cognitive model of BPD (Beck & Freeman, 1990). When asked to complete the CSQ, patients with BPD tend to identify entirely positive DOs for interpersonal interactions and tend to report AOs that they see as entirely negative. By encouraging the patient to reflect on the discrepancy between the DO and the AO, the therapist is able to challenge the patient's dichotomous thinking in a way that is nonjudgmental and tied to a concrete example.

In addition, our clinical work suggests that patients with BPD tend to hold interpretations of interpersonal encounters that are similar to the early maladaptive schemas identified by Young (1987), particularly the schemas for loss, mistrust, and guilt. The therapist is directed to attend to these when reviewing a patient's CSQ. Using the CBASP approach to treatment, these interpretations can then be challenged by questioning whether they seemed to help or hinder the patient's progress toward his or her DO. In our experience, this form of challenging is relatively non-judgmental and less likely to elicit negative reactions from the patient, compared with a more direct challenge to the rational validity of the interpretation. This form of challenging also validates the patient's experiences by allowing him or her to honestly express the thoughts that occurred during the situation, while encouraging the patient to consider revision of unhelpful interpretations. We feel that this balance is similar to the one suggested by the dialectical approach to treatment of BPD.

The second application of the CSQ occurs when the patient and therapist use it between sessions to respond to crises. Drawing inspiration from the chain analysis used in DBT, this application focuses almost exclusively on the interpretations that the patient had during a crisis and the specific behaviors in which he or she engaged. When dealing with a more dysregulated patient, the therapist is encouraged to focus more on overt behaviors, whereas with a less dysregulated patient who is better able to reflect on his or her inner state during a crisis, the therapist can focus more attention on interpretations. In this manner, the CBASP approach can help teach the relationships between the elements that escalate a crisis for the patient and help illustrate points for intervention. In the early stages of treatment, the patient and therapist may struggle together to use this application of the CSQ, but as the patient becomes more familiar with this technique, he or she should be able to apply it with greater autonomy.

The final application of the CSQ occurs when the therapist and the patient use it to understand conflicts that occur during the session. Here, the goal is to use the CSQ to highlight disruptive interpretations, behaviors, and DOs during a real-time interpersonal encounter. This is the most challenging application for the patient, who must deal with the strong emotions elicited by interpersonal conflict, and therefore it is recommended for the later stages of treatment.

CASE EXAMPLE

Ben is a 26-year-old, single, White male. He did not graduate from high school; however, he subsequently earned a general equivalency diploma (GED). He has worked a variety of jobs throughout his adult life and is currently employed through a temporary agency as an office assistant. He was referred to the clinic by a local hospital fol-

3. BORDERLINE PERSONALITY DISORDER

lowing a free mental health screening. At intake, Ben complained of a variety of symptoms, including mood swings, low self-esteem, difficulties in both family and dating relationships, anxiety and worry, guilt, substance abuse, sleep difficulties, and chronic feelings of sadness and lack of motivation. He reported suicidal ideation dating back to age 16, with at least five suicide attempts, including cutting his wrists, swallowing pills, and jumping off a two-story building. At the time of referral, Ben met *DSM–IV* criteria for BPD (American Psychiatric Association, 1994). In the initial stages of treatment, an agreement was reached between the therapist and Ben that the patient would not engage in any self-injurious or suicidal behavior. Ben agreed that if he became suicidal, he would call the therapist before he engaged in such behavior. The following transcript is from Ben's eighth therapy session; prior to this session, no suicidal gestures had been made. The course of treatment involved weekly meetings in which a completed CSQ was reviewed.

Therapist: Okay, Ben, I see that you've brought in your homework assignment for today. Why don't you go ahead and tell me about the situation that you outlined in Step 1 of the CSQ. I'm going to write it down here as you're describing it so that I can make sure that I get all of the details.

Ben: My girlfriend and I had an argument about her going back to Mexico for that missionary work that she does. When we were done arguing, I tried to hold her hand, but she said wouldn't let me because she said it's against her religion.

Therapist: Okay, let me make sure I have this right . . . First, you and Andi had an argument. Following the argument, you tried to hold her hand, but she would not allow you to do that based on her religious beliefs. Do I have that right?

Ben: Yes, that's basically what happened.

Therapist: Okay, now let's go on to Step 2. Tell me your thoughts and interpretations of that situation. One way to do this is to fill in the blank: "When I was there in that situation, it meant blank." Tell me what this situation meant to you.

Ben: Well, I thought to myself, "Why can't I show affection?"

Therapist: So, to you, holding hands would be a sign of affection.

Ben: Yeah, holding hands is a sign of affection, and what's wrong with that?

Therapist: Ok, good, that's a good one. Did you have any other interpretations?

Ben:	Yeah . . . I know she's kissing other men in Mexico.
Therapist:	Okay, you thought to yourself, "I know she's kissing other men in Mexico." What is your interpretation of that thought? What does that mean to you?
Ben:	She's cheating on me.
Therapist:	Okay, so when you were in the situation and Andi refused to hold your hand, you thought to yourself, "I know she's cheating on me in Mexico and kissing other men." Did you have any other thoughts or interpretations?
Ben:	We've kissed in the past, but everything has changed since she returned from Mexico the first time.
Therapist:	Okay, so that's good. Now we have three interpretations to work with. Let's go on to Step 3. What were your behaviors? When you tried to hold Andi's hand and she would not let you, what did you say and do in the situation?
Ben:	I told her to go and kiss her Mexican friends!
Therapist:	And how did you say that? What was your tone?
Ben:	I don't know. I just said it.
Therapist:	If I was a fly on the wall, what would I have seen and heard?
Ben:	I guess I sounded sort of sarcastic or cocky, like, fine . . . whatever . . . go kiss whomever you want. I don't care!
Therapist:	Okay, I think I can picture it. What else did you say and do?
Ben:	I turned away from her.
Therapist:	Did you say anything else?
Ben:	Well, when she got up to leave I said, "If you leave now, then it's over for good!" I also told her that if she left, I would kill myself.
Therapist:	And what was your tone when you said that?
Ben:	The same as before, I wasn't really yelling, but I was letting her know that I was angry.
Therapist:	Okay, so your tone was angry and forceful.
Ben:	Yeah, I wanted her to know that I was serious.
Therapist:	So, let me make sure I have all of this down. After you and Andi had an argument, you reached out to her and tried to hold her hand, but she would not hold your hand because she felt it was against her religious beliefs. You responded by turning away from her and telling her to go kiss her Mexican friends. When she got up to leave, you told her that if she left it would be over between you for good, and that you would kill yourself.
Ben:	Well, when you say it like that it sounds bad.
Therapist:	I'm not trying to make it sound bad or good. I just want to make sure that I have an accurate account of the facts.

3. BORDERLINE PERSONALITY DISORDER

43

Ben: Yeah, I guess that's what happened . . . but it wasn't my fault.

Therapist: No one is assigning blame here, Ben. Let's go on to Step 4 and see how this situation ended up. What was the actual outcome in this situation?

Ben: She left and I got drunk and went to the store and bought a bottle of sleeping pills.

Therapist: Did you take the pills?

Ben: No.

Therapist: What kept you from taking the pills?

Ben: I passed out before I had a chance to take them.

Therapist: So, it sounds like there were some other thoughts going on in Step 2 that we missed the first time through.

Ben: What do you mean?

Therapist: How did you get from her getting up to leave to telling her you were going to kill yourself? What were you thinking?

Ben: "If I tell her I'm going to kill myself, she'll stay."

Therapist: Let me write that down. . . . Okay, we'll come back to that in a few minutes. Before we do that, what did you want to happen? What was your desired outcome?

Ben: That she would have stayed to discuss it.

Therapist: So what you wanted was for Andi to stay and discuss what had just happened, and what actually happened was that she left without discussing it? Is that about right?

Ben: Yes.

Therapist: So you know what comes next . . . did you get what you wanted in this situation?

Ben: No!

Therapist: Okay, now let's look at each thought and interpretation to see whether it helped you or hurt you in getting your desired outcome of Andi staying to discuss the situation with you. The first thing you told me was that you thought, "Why can't I show affection." Did that thought help you or hurt you in achieving your desired outcome of Andi staying to discuss the situation?

Ben: I don't know. I don't really think it hurt.

Therapist: I'm not sure either, let's put it this way . . . do you think it helped you to get Andi to stay?

Ben: I guess not.

Therapist: I don't think so either. What do you think you could have thought instead?

Ben: I don't know . . . maybe, "I really want to show her how much I care about her."

Therapist: Good! I think that's a great thought! Can you think of any more?

Ben:	Holding hands is a sign of affection . . . I just still don't understand why we are not allowed to touch each other!
Therapist:	What could you have thought that could have helped you understand her beliefs?
Ben:	Maybe . . . I don't know, maybe I should ask her to explain her religion to me.
Therapist:	Great! It seems to me that thinking, "I really want to show her how much I care about her" and "I should ask her to explain her religion to me" would have helped you to get your desired outcome of Andi staying to discuss things with you. Now, since we're running low on time, let's look at your thoughts "I know she's cheating on me and kissing other men in Mexico" and "we've kissed in the past, but everything has changed since she returned from Mexico" together. Do you think those thoughts helped you or hurt you in achieving your desired outcome of Andi staying to discuss the situation with you.
Ben:	I think those probably hurt. They just pissed me off.
Therapist:	I agree with that. What would have been a more helpful interpretation?
Ben:	(*pause*) Maybe that's the way people greet each other in Mexico.
Therapist:	Okay, that's great! What are some other helpful thoughts?
Ben:	I trust Andi. She loves me.
Therapist:	Beautiful! It sounds to me that if you were thinking those thoughts, it definitely would have helped you to achieve your desired outcome. Now, let's look at the thought "If I tell her I'm going to kill myself, she'll stay." Do you think that one helped you or hurt you?
Ben:	I guess it hurt.
Therapist:	You don't sound convinced.
Ben:	It's just hard to give that one up.
Therapist:	I know, Ben, that's been an effective strategy for you for a long time now. But I agree with you. It didn't help you to achieve your desired outcome in this situation. What do you think you could have thought instead?
Ben:	I don't know . . . I don't think there was anything I could have thought that would really have made her stay.
Therapist:	I know this is hard. Just try to think about some helpful thoughts that may have helped you to regulate your emotions and the way you were interacting with her.
Ben:	Maybe just thinking, "I really want her to stay and talk to me."
Therapist:	That sounds good. Is there anything else?
Ben:	How about "I want us to work this out!"

3. BORDERLINE PERSONALITY DISORDER

Therapist: I think that's a great one! You are really getting better at this! I know it is hard to generate these kinds of thoughts, especially in the heat of the moment, but you are doing a great job so far, and it's only going to get easier the more we practice! Let's move on to your behaviors . . . you said that you told her, "Why don't you go kiss your Mexican friends!" I think that we can agree that that wasn't a helpful thing to say. What could you have said to help you get your desired outcome of Andi staying to talk with you?

Ben: Maybe I could have asked her to explain why she doesn't want to hold my hand . . . to explain the rules of her religion to me.

Therapist: I think that would have been a helpful thing to say. I know we're sort of rushing through this, but I think you are getting the hang of it. Let's move on to the last thing you said. "If you leave now, then it's over for good and I'm going to kill myself!" Do you think that one was helpful or hurtful?

Ben: We both know it was hurtful.

Therapist: What could you have said instead?

Ben: Andi, I just really want you to stay and talk to me!

Therapist: Good. Is there anything else?

Ben: I could have told her that I love her, I guess.

Therapist: I agree, Ben, I think that would have helped you get your desired outcome. Now, let's wrap things up . . . what have you learned from this situation?

Ben: I guess that, if I want to work things out with Andi, I need to be honest about how I feel and to be respectful to her. Threatening to kill myself is not fair to her and, at least in this situation, didn't get me what I wanted.

Therapist: Good work today. I know this isn't easy for you, but you are making a lot of progress. Keep working on these homework assignments and it's only going to get easier!

The case described here illustrates the possible use of CBASP with patients meeting criteria for BPD. Although this case was in the early stages of treatment, using the CSQ proved an effective strategy to help Ben regulate his emotions, develop effective problem-solving techniques, stabilize his interpersonal relationships, and understand the link between his interpretations and behaviors and the way people respond to him. It is important to note that following this interaction a detailed assessment of his current suicidal ideation and safety was conducted. It was determined that he was at moderate risk and a revised plan was developed to maintain his safety.

One of the inherent strengths in CBASP is its relative simplicity. The very nature of the CSQ allows for treatment of therapy-interfering behaviors, repair of rifts in the therapeutic relationship, problem solving, and skills training. In addition, using the CSQ requires the therapist to focus on acceptance and validation. The first stage of the process allows the patient to describe his or her thoughts and behaviors as they actually happened, without being judged or evaluated. The patient feels accepted and validated through the therapist listening and taking notes on the details of the situation. It is not until the remedial phase of CBASP that the therapist and the patient evaluate the effectiveness of his or her thoughts and behaviors in achieving the DO. Again, the therapist is not making judgments about the patient's thoughts and behaviors but is helping the patient to modify those that are deemed dysfunctional. As with DBT, CBASP provides a balance between acceptance and change through the use of the CSQ.

In addition, as indicated previously, throughout treatment, CSQs may be used in session as an effective way to deal with interactions between the therapist and the patient that may be interfering with the course of treatment (e.g., the patient consistently misses sessions, the therapist is pushing too hard, the patient becomes hostile).

OBSTACLES TO TREATMENT

Although CBASP is likely to provide an additional option for the effective treatment of BPD, there are certain aspects of the disorder that are likely to be obstacles to a successful outcome. Recurrent suicidal threats, gestures, and behaviors are particularly prevalent among patients with BPD (Linehan, 1993a). If, at any point in treatment, the patient is at immediate risk for harming him- or herself, the focus of therapy must shift to ensure the patient's safety. However, once the patient's safety has been established, the CSQ can be an effective tool for helping the patient develop more effective coping strategies.

In addition, there are a variety of therapy-interfering behaviors that may be obstacles to treatment. For example, the patient may fail to attend sessions on a regular basis. Obviously, it is impossible to conduct effective therapy if the patient is not attending. Additional behaviors that may interfere with therapy include refusal to work in therapy, lying, refusing to do homework, coming to sessions under the influence of drugs or alcohol,

3. BORDERLINE PERSONALITY DISORDER

and failing to work toward treatment goals and comply with the treatment contract. These behaviors are common among patients with BPD and in some cases may be diagnostic. Therefore, it is essential to establish, up front, a treatment contract and the goals for therapy. Once the patient has agreed to the contract and goals, the CSQ can be used within session, as well as on the telephone, to help the patient abandon the therapy-interfering behaviors and replace them with more adaptive, functional behaviors.

An additional obstacle is that the therapist may have a difficult time getting the patient to conform to the structure of the session. The treatment focuses on reviewing one or two CSQs in session. Therefore, it is necessary for the patient to bring in completed homework assignments to be analyzed in session. It may be difficult for patients with this disorder to complete the homework assignments outside of the session and bring one in each week. In addition, the lives of patients with BPD are often rife with interpersonal difficulties and crises. As a result, these patients often come to the session wanting to discuss the latest crisis, instead of working on the homework. In some cases, this may be appropriate; however, the therapist must be careful to be consistent in the implementation of the treatment plan and resist the urge to follow the patient's lead in all cases. Through the use of consultation, the therapist can work to follow the treatment plan, while balancing an appropriate level of crisis intervention.

Treatment for BPD is often a challenging endeavor for both therapists and patients. In the face of this challenge, several major approaches to treatment have been developed, and, among them, DBT has shown some efficacy for the treatment of this disorder. CBASP-inspired techniques, particularly the use of the CSQ, may be valuable tools for treatment. These techniques are relatively simple, compared with those associated with traditional psychoanalytic and more contemporary cognitive-behavioral approaches to treatment. This relative simplicity may offer two important advantages for treatment. For therapists, these techniques may be more easily mastered during training and executed during therapy sessions. For patients, these techniques may seem less abstruse and more problem focused. They implicitly validate the patient, model careful analysis of distressing situations, and orient the patient toward concrete strategies for future situations.

Clearly, the value of any approach to treatment is measured by its demonstrated efficacy in reducing symptoms and improving functioning in patients. For this reason, this chapter advances CBASP as a compelling avenue for evaluation by clinicians and researchers. Here again, the relative simplicity of CBASP-inspired techniques may be an important advantage. Our clinical work suggests that they can be incorporated into existing programs of therapy that are based on cognitive-behavioral or interpersonal approaches to treatment. This suggests the possibility of treatment studies that evaluate the incremental inclusion of these techniques in treatment for patients with BPD. In addition, the CSQ may offer a rich but relatively standardized data source for more fine-grained analyses of treatment mechanisms.

Chapter 4

Passive-Aggressive (Negativistic) Personality Disorder*

> Passive-Aggressive Personality Disorder is characterized by a pattern of negativistic attitudes, passive resistance to the demands of others, and negative reactivity (e.g., hostile defiance, scorning of authority). There is currently no empirically validated treatment for this disorder; however, the Cognitive Behavior Analysis System of Psychotherapy seems to be a promising new frontier in reducing these attitudes and behaviors. This chapter includes several examples of the application of Situational Analysis to the problematic thoughts and behaviors expressed by a patient with this disorder.

Passive-Aggressive Personality Disorder (PAPD) is characterized by a pervasive pattern of passive resistance and negative reactivity. *The Diagnostic and Statistical Manual of Mental Disorders–Fourth Edition (DSM–IV;* American Psychiatric Association, 1994) notes that this pattern begins by early adulthood and is present in a variety of contexts. To be diagnosed with PAPD, an individual must meet at least four of the following criteria: passive resistance to completing routine social and occupational tasks, complaints of being misunderstood and unappreciated by others, sullen or argumentative, unreasonably criticizes or scorns authority, expresses envy and resentment toward those more fortunate, exaggerated and persistent complaints of personal misfortune, and alternations between hostile defiance and contrition. If present, the criteria cannot occur exclusively during a major depressive episode and should not be better accounted for by Dysthymic Disorder.

---

*The primary authors contributing to this chapter were Mark D. Reeves and Marisol Perez.

The validity of PAPD is a matter of some controversy, and the disorder is currently listed in the appendix of the *DSM–IV* (American Psychiatric Association, 1994) as a disorder requiring further study. The diagnosis was classified as a personality disorder in earlier versions of the *DSM* but was not included in the *DSM–IV* because the authors felt that the scope of the disorder was too narrow. The *DSM–IV* committee also concluded that the PAPD diagnosis involved too few domains of functioning, displayed unacceptably high comorbidity rates with other personality disorders, and was too situational to meet the general personality disorder criterion of pervasiveness (Millon, 1993; Millon & Radovanov, 1995). Despite this criticism, there are those who argue for again including PAPD in the personality disorders section of the *DSM*. These proponents claim that the narrow breadth of PAPD is actually an asset, yielding diagnostic consistency and thus clinical use (Wetzler & Morey, 1999). Specifically, Wetzler and Morey (1999) argued that other personality disorders cannot always be reliably diagnosed due to considerable within-diagnosis heterogeneity, which does not occur in the PAPD criteria. Wetzler and Morey (1999) also observed that the comorbidity rates of PAPD are not any higher than the comorbidity rates of other personality disorders. These authors noted that all personality disorders display high comorbidity rates and concluded that it is illogical to apply a higher standard to PAPD alone. Lastly, Wetzler and Morey (1999) provided evidence that PAPD is not situation specific, arguing that patients diagnosed with PAPD display passive-aggressive behaviors in a variety of contexts, including personal relationships, work, and school. For example, a college student diagnosed with PAPD might refuse to complete a homework assignment that he or she views as unfair, might "forget" to show up for work, and might neglect to return a boyfriend's or girlfriend's phone calls. Joiner and Rudd (2002) found that the incremental validity of PAPD (defined as its ability to predict functioning controlling for all other personality disorder syndromes) exceeded that of all other personality disorder syndromes. They concluded that passive-aggressive symptoms display high validity and that PAPD, in some form, may deserve reinclusion on Axis II of future editions of *DSM*.

Regardless of this controversy, there are patients who seek treatment in clinical settings that would clearly meet the diagnostic criteria for PAPD (American Psychiatric Association, 1994). For these patients, passive-aggressive tendencies are detrimental and interfere with their interpersonal, social, and occupational functioning. Others may reject people with passive-aggressive tendencies in personal relationships or terminate them

4. PASSIVE-AGGRESSIVE PERSONALITY DISORDER

from work positions due to their oppositional behavior. If rejections and terminations become frequent, the patients' functioning may deteriorate significantly. For this reason, passive-aggressive tendencies cannot be ignored or go untreated.

HISTORY OF TREATMENT OF PAPD

Very few treatments have been developed for PAPD, and there is no empirically validated treatment for the diagnosis (Crits-Christoph, 1998). Beck and Freeman (1990) developed a cognitive approach to treating PAPD that consists of identifying and evaluating negative automatic thoughts. The cognitive distortions associated with PAPD tend to revolve around themes such as rebelling against authority and predicting negative outcomes. Often the automatic thoughts reveal the anger and rigidity that patients with PAPD experience. For example, in the case example described later in this chapter, the patient held rigidly to his belief that arbitrary authorities were forcing him to complete worthless tasks. He experienced this automatic thought frequently, and it often resulted in his feeling aggravated. This patient would often resort to seemingly passive-aggressive maneuvers, such as avoiding these tasks, to express his anger. The unfortunate result of this particular pattern was that the patient ultimately hurt himself more than the authorities.

Beck and Freeman (1990) suggested that therapists could challenge such cognitive distortions using collaborative empiricism and cost-benefit analyses to assist patients in evaluating the validity and effectiveness of their thoughts. This means that the therapist and the patient collectively evaluate both the evidence that supports the distorted belief and evidence that refutes it. In addition, the therapist helps the patient evaluate the costs and benefits of maintaining both the distorted and the potentially more adaptive beliefs. Accordingly, Beck and Freeman (1990) recommended that therapists help patients to see that passive-aggressive behaviors usually result in situational outcomes that contradict the patient's stated goal. Another aspect of Beck and Freeman's (1990) conceptualization is that PAPD patients resort to passive-aggressive strategies because they tend to have trouble expressing anger and other negative emotions directly. Thus, Beck and Freeman (1990) recommended teaching assertiveness skills to encourage patients to express themselves more clearly and directly.

MODIFICATIONS OF CBASP FOR PAPD

The five-step Cognitive Behavioral Analysis System of Psychotherapy (CBASP; McCullough, 2000) approach is ideally suited to the treatment of PAPD for a number of reasons. For example, Step 2 of the approach— *What did the situation mean to you?*—focuses the patient on the thoughts that occurred during discrete situations under analysis. This technique helps the patient identify passive-aggressive interpretations (e.g., "I don't have to do what authorities tell me!") that were made during specific situations. Identification of these thoughts and interpretations is helpful because PAPD patients may not have been aware of them or how frequently they occur. Patients also may not know how their passive-aggressive thoughts lead to both passive-aggressive behaviors and unfavorable situational outcomes. Step 2 of CBASP illustrates these connections explicitly, thereby yielding even greater use when the therapist helps the patient to reflect back on a series of analyses of various situations. The therapist is then able to point out the frequent recurrence of certain passive-aggressive thoughts and make generalized conclusions about how such thoughts typically lead to passive-aggressive behaviors and negative situational outcomes.

Likewise, Step 3 of CBASP—*What did you do in the situation?*—helps patients to identify patterns of passive-aggressive behaviors and to recognize how these behaviors lead to negative results. This step is especially well suited to PAPD because passive behaviors may not be readily apparent to the patient or even to others with whom they interact. Specifically, it is often what the patient is not doing that is of more significance than what they are doing. Though this point may seem oversimplified, comprehending this pattern can be a very profound experience for PAPD patients. It may seem overly obvious to ask patients whether their inaction helped them to get what they wanted—the Desired Outcome (DO) in Step 4—yet it is precisely this question that creates a feeling of disharmony in patients and that ultimately motivates them to change their behavior to more active approaches. Patients cannot help but see how their lack of action may be hindering them from reaching their goals. The CBASP approach rests on the assumption that as patients repeatedly make this type of connection over several Situational Analyses (SAs), they become increasingly motivated to reduce the uncomfortable feeling that accompanies it.

4. PASSIVE-AGGRESSIVE PERSONALITY DISORDER 53

These realizations are often made during the elicitation phase of CBASP, which helps patients with PAPD to understand that their passive-aggressive thoughts and behaviors are actually quite ineffectual. In the remediation phase of CBASP, on the other hand, therapists direct their patients to generate alternative thoughts and behaviors that are more helpful in achieving their DOs than the passive-aggressive thoughts and behaviors that they used routinely before seeking treatment. This aspect of the CBASP approach provides an excellent opportunity for PAPD patients to learn new thoughts and behaviors that will improve their quality of life. Repeated experiences with the remediation phase of CBASP should encourage PAPD patients to increasingly apply alternative thoughts and behaviors to situations outside session, ultimately enabling them to change their characteristically passive-aggressive strategies.

Insofar as CBASP seems well suited to the treatment of PAPD, therapists need not modify the technique much for patients presenting with these personality features. However, there are a few issues that are worth considering with this patient population. First, therapists should direct the patient to describe situations (Step 1) in which he or she was asked to meet some reasonable request and failed to do so. During Step 2 of CBASP, therapists should probe for, and pay special attention to, the negative automatic thoughts that Beck and Freeman (1990) associated with PAPD. These include thoughts of rebellion, being misunderstood, and the arbitrary requests of authorities. As mentioned previously, analysis at Step 3 usually reveals behaviors such as inactivity, procrastination, and other passive maneuvers that are designed to express hostility indirectly. The therapist should highlight these behaviors for PAPD patients during SA.

Lastly, the therapist should be aware that a PAPD patient's DO is typically to complete some task or fulfill some request, though the patient may initially state some other goal, such as refusing to comply with seemingly unreasonable demands. In addition, the therapist may need to emphasize that although reaching specific situation-bound goals of compliance may seem demeaning and unreasonable, completing these short-term goals is often necessary for the patient to obtain the DO. Patients with PAPD features often demonstrate considerable difficulty in completing requests to achieve their DOs during the initial sessions of treatment. This difficulty likely stems from the fact that such behaviors contradict their strongly held resentment of authority. If these problems occur, the therapist should encourage the patient to hang in there, reminding the patient that learning any new skill takes time and a great deal of practice. The therapist may also need to highlight repeatedly that although compliance may seem distasteful, the patient must decide whether compliance is more distasteful than failing to achieve DOs (i.e., cost-benefit analysis).

In the remediation phase of Step 2, therapists should encourage patients to replace negative thoughts with thoughts that emphasize completing tasks that they may not find enjoyable but which they must complete to obtain some greater DO. In addition, remediation of behaviors at Step 3 should emphasize the use of assertive communication and efficient completion of tasks.

In the case of patients presenting with PAPD features, it is especially important for therapists to explain the rationale for using the Coping Survey Questionnaire (CSQ; McCullough, 2000) and illustrate how it can prove helpful to patients' presenting problems. Therapists also should make clear that the format of the CSQ provides an organized and consistent way to view situations and increases the likelihood that the patient will get what they want out of a specific situation. Providing such rationales can diminish some of the characteristic resistance to a seemingly imposed structure, which PAPD patients may exhibit when encountering the CSQ. In addition, as patients with PAPD features can be oppositional and often seek the path of least resistance, it is important for the therapist to be consistent in adhering to the CSQ format and in all other aspects of the therapeutic relationship. This means that if a patient "forgets" to complete CSQ homework or attempts to steer conversation away from the situation being examined, the therapist must address the noncompliance directly and assertively or steer conversation back to SA.

CASE EXAMPLE

Jeremy was a 24-year-old student who reported experiencing a 4-month major depressive episode during his 1st year of graduate school. He reported that he remained isolated in his house for much of this time and rarely attended classes, ultimately resulting in his expulsion from his program. However, after some discussions with faculty, Jeremy was granted a second chance. In intake sessions at our clinic, Jeremy was described as angry, argumentative, and sometimes lacking empathy.

4. PASSIVE-AGGRESSIVE PERSONALITY DISORDER

Though initially it appeared that Jeremy's primary diagnoses were Major Depressive Disorder and Narcissistic Personality Disorder, later reexamination of his case suggested the possibility of PAPD. In particular, Jeremy's tendencies to resent authorities and see them as arbitrary, procrastinate on assigned tasks, make many false starts without completion, and express resentment and anger through passive-aggressive behaviors strongly implicated PAPD.

Jeremy reported several previous treatment experiences during the intake interview, most of them quite negative (e.g., he recalled a therapist he saw as a child whom he felt forced him to decide with which parent he wanted to live). It could be argued that by relating these negative impressions during his first session, Jeremy appeared to be communicating to the therapist that he was wary of psychologists and thus might be on the defensive.

Fortunately, Jeremy had recently had a positive experience with a counselor after he was arrested for an offense related to substance abuse. Jeremy attributed his comfort to this counselor's down-to-earth and humble approach. Jeremy noted that since the counselor had suffered from substance-related problems, Jeremy viewed him less as a cold authority and more as a warm, understanding human being.

Jeremy attended just over 20 sessions at our clinic. Much of his therapy was directed toward the treatment of symptoms associated with NPD, Major Depressive Disorder (MDD), and Generalized Anxiety Disorder (GAD). The therapist used elements of Beck's cognitive therapies for NPD and MDD and Barlow's treatment for GAD for the first several sessions. CBASP was only used systematically to specifically target Jeremy's passive-aggressive symptoms for the last seven sessions. This was due in part to initial doubt about whether PAPD was a suitable, primary diagnosis for Jeremy. Although he ultimately terminated against the therapist's advice, Jeremy made substantial progress during sessions in which the therapist used CBASP. Although the therapist only used the CSQ for seven sessions, Jeremy clearly learned during this time that his thoughts and behaviors were key to his repeated frustration in achieving DOs and yet also held the potential to bringing those outcomes within reach. This was clearly the most productive therapy experience of Jeremy's life.

TABLE 4.1
CSQ Illustrating Jeremy's Passive-Aggressive Pattern
of Thoughts and Behaviors

Step 1 Situation	• I sat down to do my homework. • I thought about how unfair the assignment was. • I decided to do other things.
Step 2 Interpretations	• This assignment is unfair because it requires a special program only available on campus that I can't download for use at home. • I shouldn't have to do this assignment. • There is no value to me for doing this assignment. • I'm being made to do something I don't want to do.
Step 3 Behaviors	• Sat down to do homework • Got up to do something else
Step 4 Desired outcome	• To complete my homework
Step 5 Outcome	• Did not complete my homework
Step 6 Comparison of Actual and Desired Outcomes	• Did not get what I wanted

When completing CSQs with Jeremy, the focus was on his tendency to avoid working on homework in certain classes. Table 4.1 presents a CSQ from one session with Jeremy and what follows is a partial transcript of the session.

Therapist: Okay! So, we know that you have had this assignment a long time and that it's overdue. How about we look at one time when you were working on the assignment?

Jeremy: Well, a couple nights ago I finally sat down at my desk and looked at the assignment. I spent a couple hours trying to get a free copy of the stupid computer program we have to use, and I couldn't find it on the Internet. The whole assignment is a waste of time because it's nothing like what I'll actually be doing.

Therapist: Okay, I wrote that you sat down to do your homework and decided it was unfair. What else happened in the situation?

Jeremy: (*silent, staring intensely at the therapist*) I didn't do it.

Therapist: Okay. You didn't do it. So you did something else instead, right?

Jeremy: Yeah. I went and watched TV.

4. PASSIVE-AGGRESSIVE PERSONALITY DISORDER 57

Therapist: That's Step 1. We made a very brief, bulleted description of the situation. Now let's go to Step 2. What did the situation mean to you? What were you thinking?

Jeremy: I was thinking how stupid the assignment was. I couldn't understand why I had to go and use this program when there are other more common programs that I would actually use in real life. I was thinking this assignment was useless to me since it's artificial and doesn't relate to my work. Overall, I was thinking that I was being forced to do something that I really didn't want to do.

Therapist: Okay. Got that down. That's Step 2, your thoughts. Now let's go to Step 3, your behaviors. What did you do in the situation? It sounds like you sat down to do your homework, didn't do your homework, then got up to do something else. What did you want in the situation?

Jeremy: To finish the assignment.

Therapist: How did things turn out in the situation?

Jeremy: What do you mean?

Therapist: What was the end result of the situation, the outcome?

Jeremy: I didn't do my homework.

Therapist: Okay, so like we said before: You don't like this assignment, but you know it will help you pass this class so you won't get kicked out of your program again. Did you get what you wanted?

Jeremy: (*long silence: stares intensely at ground, then at therapist*) No.

Therapist: Now, let's look back at your thoughts and behaviors to see if they were helpful or hurtful. Did thinking to yourself, "This assignment is unfair because it requires a special program only available on campus that I can't download for use at home" help you or hurt you to get the assignment done?

Jeremy: I guess it didn't help.

Therapist: Makes sense. If you feel the assignment is unfair, you'd probably feel kinda upset and not want to do the thing. How about the other thoughts, "I shouldn't have to do the assignment," "There is no value to me for doing this assignment," and "I'm being made to do something I don't want to do." Did those help or hurt?

Jeremy: They didn't help. They just made me more pissed off at this stupid assignment.

Therapist: Okay. How about your behaviors? Did sitting down at the table help?

Jeremy: No.

Therapist: Well, okay. But, at least you're sitting down to work on it, right? Instead of totally avoiding your desk?

Jeremy:	I guess.
Therapist:	So, that's a tough one, but I'd say it actually helped. How about getting up to do something else?
Jeremy:	Obviously that didn't help.
Therapist:	Right. Let's go back over this situation to see if you could have thought or done anything differently to get what you wanted. So, what else could you have thought to get what you wanted? Again, I'm not trying to tell you what you should want, and I'm not arguing that you have to do what other people want. I'm assuming that you wanted to get the assignment done. What else could you have thought?
Jeremy:	(*silence*) I don't know. I didn't want to do it.
Therapist:	Okay, how about "I really don't want to do this stupid assignment, but I have to if I want to pass this stupid class. I guess I'd better just do the stupid thing so I can move on."
Jeremy:	(*laughs*) Yeah, I guess that would help. But it's hard to think those things. I know I should think them, but I don't. I keep thinking how stupid the assignment is.
Therapist:	That's totally normal, and it's why you're here. Listen, if you practice this thing we're doing, you will eventually come to think and do things that will at least help you get what you want in every situation, at every moment in your life. The thoughts here on the paper are knee-jerk for you. You automatically think them every time you get what you see as a dumb assignment. If you keep practicing the helpful thoughts, though, they will hopefully become automatic and replace the hurtful thoughts. Okay, now let's look at your behavior.
Jeremy:	Well that's obvious. Not doing the homework didn't help me do the homework.
Therapist:	Yeah, this stuff is kind of commonsense, but it helps to really look at what you're doing in each situation to see if it's helping you or hurting you. Well, okay. So what else could you have done?
Jeremy:	Just do the damn assignment.
Therapist:	Yeah . . . I think that would help. (*smiles*)
Jeremy:	You know, I have all these different thoughts. I think about trying to change the system. I think about what else I could be doing. I think about what I'd do if I were in charge. I wonder if things from my past are making me not do this stuff. I'm not sure what the right thing is to think!
Therapist:	Yeah, we could come up with all kinds of ways of looking at this, right? We could come up with lots of different theories and spec-

4. PASSIVE-AGGRESSIVE PERSONALITY DISORDER

ulate about why you do these things. You know what, though? It really comes down to one simple question: Does it help or does it hurt? Is thinking this helping me to get what I want, or hurting me?

As can be seen from this transcript, Jeremy's interpretations from Step 2 were actually quite similar to those described by Beck and Freeman (1990) as characteristic of those with PAPD symptoms and seemingly led Jeremy to refuse to comply with demands that he perceived as unfair and coming from arbitrary authorities. The end result, however, was to take Jeremy one step closer to again being expelled from his program. He stated that he wanted to complete the program, which now required obtaining a high grade in all of his classes to make up for his poor grades. Examining the thoughts and behaviors Jeremy chose in this situation revealed that none of them helped him to complete his homework, and all of them hurt him in achieving this DO. However, Jeremy was able to understand that choosing other thoughts and behaviors could help him achieve his DO.

Jeremy's pattern of passive-aggressive behavior was apparent in his behavior with the therapist (see Table 4.2). At first, Jeremy arrived late

TABLE 4.2
CSQ Illustrating Jeremy's Passive-Aggressive Pattern
with the Therapist

Step 1 Situation	• I came to session without the book.
Step 2 Interpretations	• I don't have to bring the book. • There will be no negative consequences for not bringing the book. • I don't have to do what my therapist tells me.
Step 3 Behaviors	• I left home without the book.
Step 4 Desired outcome	• Bring the book to therapy
Step 5 Outcome	• I arrived at therapy without the book.
Step 6 Comparison of Actual and Desired Outcomes	• Did not get what I wanted

to session on several occasions. He explained that he was running late for class and denied any aggressive motives. Later, the therapist lent Jeremy a book, and Jeremy forgot to bring the book for five consecutive sessions. Jeremy again denied any motive for this behavior and repeatedly promised to bring the book at the following session. The therapist finally confronted Jeremy with the possibility that these behaviors were in fact part of a passive-aggressive pattern of resisting external demands. The following CSQ was the result of the therapist's prompting Jeremy to look for the passive-aggressive thoughts he had regarding returning the book. The following transcript elaborates the details of the discussion.

Jeremy: I forgot the book again. I'm really sorry.

Therapist: Hmm. I have an idea. I wonder if you're trying to tell me something by not bringing the book. I wonder if this is part of the passive-aggressive pattern we've been talking about.

Jeremy: Really, I just forgot it. There's nothing more to it.

Therapist: Hypothetically, what might you be angry with me about?

Jeremy: Look, there's really nothing to this. I just keep forgetting the book.

Therapist: Well, that's the thing. You've forgotten it four, five times now. I have a hunch that this is an example of passive aggression.

Jeremy: I really don't know why you're insisting on this. Why don't you just drop it? I apologized.

Therapist: Okay. I know you forgot it. But we're more likely to forget certain things. For instance, if you had tickets to a concert of your favorite rock group, how likely would you be to forget the concert?

Jeremy: Hell, no. I wouldn't forget that. You couldn't stop me from getting there.

Therapist: Okay. Well, but what about a meeting of a group that you really feel is a waste of your time but that you said you'd make. Do you think it's possible that you'd be more likely to forget certain things, even though your ability to remember things is really intact? It seems that people may remember things they want to remember and forget things they want to forget.

Jeremy: Yeah, but I really do feel sorry for forgetting the book, and I really do intend to bring it. There's really no hidden agenda here. Why are you pushing me? I feel like you're making me do something I don't want to do!

Therapist: I'm trying to dig a little deeper here because I think there's something to this. I wonder if you might really be angry with

4. PASSIVE-AGGRESSIVE PERSONALITY DISORDER 61

	me and are trying to communicate this anger indirectly by not bringing the book.
Jeremy:	Well, I can see that. It makes sense.
Therapist:	Okay. So let's try again. What do you think you might be angry with me about?
Jeremy:	(*long silence*) You know, I'm never really sure if you're acting in my best interest. I never really know what you're doing, and sometimes I wonder if you're just playing with my mind for your own enjoyment. On the other hand, I don't want to ask you about this because it may be that the treatment only works if I don't really know what you're doing. Maybe it would stop working if you told me everything you are doing.
Therapist:	Ahh, that's interesting! Okay. So you would like me to be more clear with you about what I'm doing and why. I think that's totally fair and it's actually what cognitive-behavioral therapists are supposed to do. I believe that it's perfectly okay and actually quite helpful if you know what I'm doing, why I'm doing it, and how it should help. So you were just assertive with me right then. You told me flat out about something you were kind of pissed about! How did that feel?
Jeremy:	Okay. I mean, I'm assertive. I speak up against people when I think they're doing something really wrong. Like that racist boss I told you about. I told him off!
Therapist:	Yes. You were assertive then. But that was kind of an extreme case. What about when it's something more minor that kind of has you miffed, and you're not really sure about saying some-thing about it? How about we do a CSQ about this situation? The situation is that you came to session without the book. What were you thinking?
Jeremy:	I don't know.
Therapist:	Take a minute. We're not in a rush.
Jeremy:	(*silence*) Well, I guess I was thinking that there's no conse-quence.
Therapist:	What do you mean?
Jeremy:	Well, it's not like I'm going to get in trouble if I forget the book. You don't have any control over me.
Therapist:	Okay, I'll write that down. What about your behaviors? I'll just write that you didn't bring the book. What did you want?
Jeremy:	I guess I wanted to bring the book. I didn't get that.
Therapist:	Okay. What else could you have thought and done?
Jeremy:	I guess I could have thought that it's really not that hard to find the book. I could have found it and brought it.

Therapist: That's fair. You know, you're right. It's not like the world will come to an end if you don't bring it. I have no control over you. But that's a different issue than simply what you want. It sounds like you wanted to return the book.

Jeremy: Look. I'll bring it next time.

Therapist: Okay. (Jeremy brought the book to the next session.)

Note again that the thoughts and behaviors Jeremy displayed in this situation are very similar to those described by Beck and Freeman's (1990) description of PAPD symptomatology. Recall that one of Beck's formulations about people with passive-aggressive features is that they have difficulty being assertive. Working within this framework, the therapist suggested that there might be something that Jeremy was trying to communicate to the therapist indirectly by forgetting to bring the book so many times. Jeremy was defensive about this suggestion at first. Nonetheless, the therapist suggested that for Jeremy to practice changing his behavior from passive aggression to active assertion, Jeremy would have to identify why he was angry with the therapist and communicate this directly. After the therapist gave this rationale, Jeremy eventually revealed that he believed the therapist was trying to manipulate his mind in devious ways for his own pleasure.

This therapeutic breakthrough moved Jeremy from indirect communication to direct assertion. However, the encounter also revealed the first of many paranoid personality features that Jeremy eventually disclosed and which the therapist was ultimately not able to address due to Jeremy's unilateral termination from treatment. Thus, as both the critics and supporters of the PAPD diagnosis have agreed, patients who display one constellation of disordered personality features almost always display features from other personality disorders. At the least, features of PAPD, NPD, and Paranoid Personality Disorder were apparent in Jeremy's presentation. Importantly, though, his therapist might not have uncovered the paranoid features if he had ignored Jeremy's passive-aggressive personality features. This anecdotal evidence provides more support for the place of PAPD in the psychiatric nosology.

As Beck and Freeman (1990) note, it is best practice for therapists treating passive-aggressive patients to be completely explicit in explaining the treatment and rationale, even more so than is standard practice in cognitive-behavioral therapy. In fact, Jeremy responded well when the therapist began to explain every move he made in session. For example, the therapist would preface a discussion of the evidence for and against a thought with the following: "I'd like to take a look at the thought you just mentioned by coming up with evidence that supports the thought and evidence that goes against the thought. I think that looking at this evidence would help you decide whether the thought is realistic and ultimately decide whether the thought is helping you or hurting you in getting things you want out of the situation. Is that okay with you?" Providing these kinds of explanations is vital when using the CBASP approach with PAPD patients. In the absence of specific rationales, such patients are likely to view the approach as simply another authoritarian structure imposed by an arbitrary authority—the therapist. Transparency also makes the therapist appear like less of an authority and more of a human being who is sharing a helpful solution.

Outcome

Although Jeremy seemed to appreciate this more explicit approach, he ultimately terminated therapy against the advice of the therapist. He called to explain that he had decided to drop out of school and could no longer afford therapy. The therapist felt it was important to have a formal termination session with Jeremy to attempt to change his pattern of ending relationships passively, which he had reported during treatment. After several weeks of failed attempts at scheduling a termination session with Jeremy, the therapist decided it was better to terminate with Jeremy by phone than to have no termination at all. He reached Jeremy at home and explained that he felt it was in Jeremy's best interest to have a formal termination so that this therapeutic episode would end in an active and clear way.

Jeremy agreed and listened as the therapist reviewed the content and process of his course of treatment and mentioned his perceptions of Jeremy's strengths and weaknesses. The therapist explained what he had learned from Jeremy, such as the importance of explicitly explaining and giving a rationale for treatments, and made recommendations in the event that Jeremy decided to reinitiate treatment in the future. Lastly, the therapist stated that Jeremy was welcome to return to the clinic at any time.

OBSTACLES TO TREATMENT

As with the case example, the most common obstacle encountered when conducting therapy with PAPD patients is resistance. When patients passively refuse to complete reasonable and agreed-upon therapeutic tasks in session, the therapist can use CBASP or motivational interviewing techniques (Miller & Rollnick, 2002) to evaluate the effectiveness of the patient's passive behavior in reaching his or her own stated goals for therapy. For example, the therapist can guide the patient through a consideration of the pros and cons of actively engaging in therapy.

A related common obstacle with this patient population is failure to complete homework assignments. If a patient comes to session without having completed assigned CSQ homework tasks, the therapist should emphasize that the patient will reach goals more quickly if he or she completes homework regularly. The therapist should then proceed to complete a CSQ in session on either the failure to complete homework or some situation from the previous week.

When they do complete CSQ homework assignments, patients with PAPD features often initially exhibit characteristic problems in learning the method. For example, a common problem for these patients involves Step 1, describing the situation. In Step 1, the patient is to provide only objective facts related to the event and avoid emotionally laden descriptions. However, PAPD patients may have a hard time distinguishing thoughts from emotions and understanding that particular thoughts contribute to certain emotional experiences. It often takes patients with PAPD several sessions of completing CSQs before they understand the distinction between thoughts and emotions. Learning this difference, however, enhances the patient's ability to organize information during stressful situations and facilitates subsequent thought analysis.

PAPD patients may also have difficulty with Step 5 of the CSQ, describing how the situation turned out. In completing their first few CSQs, these patients often fail to notice the emotional consequences that result from failing to obtain their DOs. They have difficulty understanding that failing to get what they want can lead to feelings of sadness, anger, or guilt, which can compound any comorbid mood and anxiety disorders. For example, when Jeremy described the outcome of the situation in which he failed to return the book, he neglected to comment on any feelings of guilt he might have experienced as a result of not complying with his therapist's simple request. Thus, Jeremy's interpretations indicate that he believed that there were no consequences to his forgetting the book. Although there might not have been any externally observable consequences to his inaction, failing to return the book likely caused unpleasant emotions that Jeremy failed to identify. If patients with PAPD features display this kind of difficulty, therapists should explicitly make the connection between failing to get one's DO and resultant negative emotions, in arguably an undesirable outcome. Such interventions can help PAPD patients understand how their pattern of passive aggression can maintain comorbid disorders, such as depression. In Jeremy's case, it seems plausible to conclude that consequences associated with his passive-aggressive personality features contributed to his 4-month depressive episode.

It is important to remember several things when implementing CBASP with patients presenting with PAPD features. First, the CSQ is used within the cognitive framework of Beck and Freeman's (1990) conceptualization of PAPD to identify characteristic negative automatic thoughts and replace them with more effective thoughts. Second, PAPD patients tend to resist treatment or homework assignments, such as the CSQ. When this occurs, the therapist can actually complete a CSQ on the patients' resistance to do their homework, as when the therapist in the case example used the CSQ to understand why Jeremy would not return a book the therapist lent him. Third, it is especially important to keep a collaborative stance with patients with PAPD features and provide an explicit rationale for all therapeutic interventions. Last, it should be noted that use of the CSQ not only can help reduce passive-aggressive tendencies but also can address other conditions such as depression and anxiety that often cooccur with PAPD.

As noted previously, CBASP is ideally suited to treating PAPD. The treatment effectively uncovers passive-aggressive thoughts and behaviors that may not be readily apparent to the patient or to others. CBASP also uniquely highlights how such thoughts and behaviors are counterproductive through repeated evaluations of their effectiveness in achieving situational DOs. Lastly, a therapist using CBASP is able to assist patients diagnosed with PAPD in generating and practicing active thoughts and assertive behaviors. In the context of a warm, transparent therapeutic relationship, CBASP offers a promising solution to this insidious personality disorder. The end result is that PAPD patients can become active participants in life, able to obtain directly and assertively that which they truly desire.

Chapter 5

Personality Disorder Not Otherwise Specified*

Personality Disorder Not Otherwise Specified is the diagnostic label applied to patients who present with a combination of the pathological personality symptoms that comprise the other personality disorders. These symptoms may also include more than one personality disorder cluster (i.e., odd/eccentric, anxious, or dramatic/erratic). This chapter presents the Cognitive Behavioral Analysis System of Psychotherapy as a method of treating the multifaceted presentations that make up this disorder. A case example describes the implementation of Situational Analysis for a patient with Personality Disorder Not Otherwise Specified with Avoidant and Schizotypal features. Obstacles to treatment, as well as possible methods of resolution, are presented.

There are few empirically validated treatments available for personality disorders, which leaves clinicians grappling with decisions on how to best treat these patients. For patients with Personality Disorder Not Otherwise Specified (PD NOS; American Psychiatric Association, 1994), treatment decisions can be even more complicated due to the presence of different combinations of symptoms from several personality disorders. This chapter focuses on the treatment of patients with PD NOS using the Cognitive Behavioral Analysis System of Psychotherapy (CBASP; McCullough, 2000) technique, modifications to the technique, obstacles to treatment, and a case example.

---

*The primary authors contributing to this chapter were Therese Skubic Kemper, Annya Hernandez, and Leonardo Bobadilla.

Personality disorders are among the most pernicious mental illnesses, given their nature as long-standing, ingrained patterns of behavior that are often resistant to treatment and the high rates of comorbidity with Axis I disorders (Crits-Christoph, 1998). The clinical picture is perhaps more complicated for PD NOS. PD NOS not only shares the previously mentioned characteristics of other, better delineated personality disorders, but it also is often complicated by vexing combinations of pathological personality symptoms from more than one personality disorder cluster (i.e., odd/eccentric, dramatic/erratic, or anxious/dependent). This variability in symptom expression makes it impractical to develop a treatment strategy specific to each combination of symptoms.

TREATMENT OF PD NOS

Even as research on the treatment of Axis I disorders continues to grow and treatment options become more effective, there remain few empirically validated treatments for personality disorders, with the exception of Dialectical Behavior Therapy (DBT) for Borderline Personality Disorder (Linehan, Hubert, Suarez, Douglas, & Heard, 1991). The paucity of research on the treatment of personality disorders has left clinicians grappling with treatment decisions and choosing treatments that have not been empirically validated. Some have suggested that research on the treatment of personality disorders should proceed in the direction of matching patients to treatment modalities based on their personality syndrome (Barber & Muenz, 1996) or salient patient variables that are not necessarily symptoms of the personality disorder (e.g., external coping style, resistance; Beutler, Mohr, Grawe, & Engel, 1991). Although these alternatives may be feasible directions for research on the treatment of specific personality disorders, it is more difficult to delineate groups of personality symptoms or patient attributes for a group of patients with PD NOS because their symptoms often fall into several diagnostic categories.

MODIFICATION OF CBASP FOR PD NOS

CBASP and the Coping Survey Questionnaire (CSQ) offer treatment strategies that need not fundamentally differ depending on the personality syndrome or specific symptoms. Though patients with well-delineated dis-

5. PERSONALITY DISORDER NOT OTHERWISE SPECIFIED

orders, such as Major Depressive Disorder or Panic Disorder, are likely to present with a core set of symptoms per the particular disorder, patients with PD NOS may appear completely symptomatically distinct from one another. Despite this circumstance, the structure and process of the CSQ remains relatively constant across clinical presentations, allowing for adaptation of the content to address problem areas specific to each individual. Therefore, thoughts and behaviors specific to each individual's symptom presentation may be targeted as points of intervention.

This adaptation enables the use of CBASP in the treatment of symptoms that are specific to particular types of features of PD NOS. For example, the treatment for patients presenting with paranoid or schizotypal features could focus on thoughts and behaviors associated with unsubstantiated paranoia and suspicion of others. Similarly, treatment focusing on the thoughts and behaviors associated with poor impulse control would be appropriate for patients diagnosed with PD NOS with antisocial or borderline features. Likewise, CBASP treatment for a patient diagnosed as having PD NOS with dependent features can center on the thoughts and behaviors associated with unrealistic fears of abandonment. Dysfunctional preoccupation with perfectionism, a feature specific to PD NOS with obsessive-compulsive features, can also be a focus of CBASP treatment.

⤳ CASE EXAMPLE ↶

Sam was a 28-year-old White male who sought treatment for problems of loneliness, social isolation, and feelings of sadness that were interfering with his motivation, energy level, and ability to concentrate, causing him to fall behind in his graduate school program. At the time of the intake interview, Sam's thought process and speech content were logical and coherent; however, he frequently did not answer questions directly and spoke philosophically and in the abstract. Sam reported that he could not remember a time during which he felt a social connection with others, even as a child, and reported never having close friends or a romantic relationship. He spoke frequently of his desire for intimate social relationships but reported social anxiety and a fear of negative evaluation by others that inhibited fulfilling this desire. Sam also expressed a simultaneous disinterest in social interactions due to the immorality and character flaws in those he was likely to encounter. Specifically, Sam found negative emotions, such as sadness, anger, and sexuality, intolerable in himself and others and felt extreme guilt as a result of the presence of these emotions. As a result, Sam forbade himself from expressing them outwardly and rarely made efforts to interact socially for fear that he might find these emotions in others. Sam often stated that he strived to reach a more enlightened and moral state in which he would be free from anger, sexuality, and sadness.

Sam was initially diagnosed with Dysthymic Disorder, and a diagnosis on Axis II was deferred. Later, a diagnosis of PD NOS with Avoidant and Schizotypal Features was given on Axis II. His Global Assessment of Functioning rating was 43 at intake. Sam's therapeutic goals included reduction of dysthymic symptoms, development of social skills, and emotional regulation focused on increasing awareness of and comfort with emotions he labeled as negative. The primary treatment approach was CBASP. Forty-six CSQ forms were completed in session, and he completed several per week on his own.

Initially, Sam expressed skepticism at the treatment approach; however, from the first session, he consistently completed homework assignments. Significant difficulties encountered during sessions included problems staying focused on the event described in the CSQ, difficulty generating specific thoughts and behaviors related to the event, difficulty generating thoughts not philosophically oriented or abstract, and difficulty generating Desired Outcomes (DOs) that did not conflict with his morals. Often, Sam found himself stating two DOs that he believed conflicted. For example, one pair of DOs was "I want to look at an attractive girl," which he saw as immoral, and "I want to be considerate toward others." Another pair of DOs was "I want to avoid a negative display of emotion" and "I want to express myself [because I was angry that I was being charged for a cancelled session]."

Sam also had difficulty generating DOs because he felt that if he did not attain what he wanted in a situation, it was because he did not truly desire it, not because of what he thought or did. His recurrent explanation of this was "My beliefs create my reality." According to Sam, this statement implied that he held beliefs, desires, and ideas that ultimately governed the outcome of situations, regardless of what he stated he wanted.

As a result of these obstacles encountered early in treatment, much of the initial work in completing the CSQ was in generating specific and concrete thoughts, behaviors, and DOs. For instance, Sam practiced changing thoughts such as, "I hypothesize that there is a part of me that wants to be close to someone and another part of me that doesn't let myself get close to someone because the usual series of events is a sort of 'split decision'" to "I thought I should ask her out, but I was nervous." Sam also practiced changing DOs such as "I want to successfully achieve my desires," "I want to successfully confront my fears," and "I want to behave in a manner that signifies that I have resolved my internal conflicts" to situation-specific goals, which included "I want to show up for my appointment," "I want to spend some casual time with friends," and "I want to express my anger in a way that does not hurt anyone."

Similar obstacles were encountered when the therapist encouraged Sam to replace hurtful thoughts and behaviors with helpful thoughts and behaviors. One obstacle was that Sam wanted to change his underlying beliefs before changing his thoughts and behaviors. His rationale for this was if he replaced his automatic thoughts and behaviors while still maintaining his beliefs and values, which he often believed conflicted, he would be deceiving himself and others. For instance, he often decided not to approach a woman to start a conversation because he was nervous, and he believed this reflected that he did not truly want to interact with her. After approximately 4 months of treatment, Sam acknowledged that his current thought and behavior patterns were not helping him meet his goals. Therefore, he decided to make attempts at generating "simple" thoughts, such as "I want to say 'hello' to her," challenging the idea that his feelings of anxiety reflected that he did not desire a particular outcome. Due to these efforts, Sam began to spontaneously generate specific, concrete, and simple thoughts as well as DOs after an additional month of treatment.

In conjunction with this practice, two particular themes of thoughts and behaviors were addressed on a regular basis during the course of completing the CSQ: those related to social anxiety and avoidance and those that were odd and abstract. Specifically, his fear of rejection was evident in many thoughts and was targeted by developing social skills to help prevent rejection, developing skills to help accurately determine whether he was truly rejected, and challenging thoughts related to the severity of the consequences if, in fact, he was truly rejected. The latter strategy was essential to Sam's discovery that the actual consequences were not as dire as he had imagined, giving him newfound confidence and the desire to pursue social contact. This, in turn, enabled him to practice social skills and gain experience in social settings, thereby decreasing the frequency of true social rejections.

Sam's abstract and philosophical thoughts were seen as an important point of intervention because they often prevented the formation of concrete and logical connections between his thoughts, emotions, and behaviors. These thoughts were targeted through a combination of approaches. First, due to the structure of the CSQ, Sam was not required to challenge the validity of his philosophical thoughts; he only needed to determine whether the thoughts helped or hurt him in achieving his DO. This was a key advantage for Sam because challenging beliefs he held dear was deemed very problematic. After several months of treatment, Sam was able to acknowledge that many of his thoughts did not help him achieve his outcomes, and some of them hurt by eliciting anxiety or leading him to act in a manner contrary to the DO. Second, when Sam generated abstract or philosophical thoughts, he was asked, "What does that look like in this particular situation?" or "What did that mean, specifically, when you were in the situation?" This led Sam to produce more concrete thoughts that were directly related to his behaviors. These thoughts, in turn, helped him discover that instead of becoming overwhelmed or anxious as a result of these thoughts, he could relate them to his behaviors and change the behaviors directly to attain his DO. Third, Sam was responsive to encouragement by his therapist to practice these strategies despite his skepticism and discomfort and made much progress due to his willingness to employ strategies with which he did not immediately agree or understand. These aspects to therapy, in combination, led to Sam's spontaneous formation of more concrete and specific DOs. As Sam became better able to specify desired goals, as well as the thoughts and behaviors that would help him achieve them, he reported feeling more in control of his environment. He began attending classes on a more regular basis to achieve his DO of passing them. His willingness to interact socially also increased, and, as a result, he began developing a social network and forming friendships.

Although positive emotional experiences accompanied these improvements, Sam was faced with his and others' troublesome negative emotions on a more regular basis. For example, he found himself

5. PERSONALITY DISORDER NOT OTHERWISE SPECIFIED

becoming frustrated with others' inconsideration, he felt angry and sad when he was rejected after requesting a date, and he continued to grapple with his discomfort with sexual desires. Sam's discomfort with these emotions then became a therapeutic focus, incorporated into the CSQ. After several weeks of discussing social norms regarding the expression of these emotions and allowing Sam to rehearse them in session, he began to practice them on his own and incorporate his experiences into the CSQ. Specifically, Sam practiced emotional regulation (i.e., anger management, self-reminders that intense emotions would subside) and engaged in more socially appropriate expressions of anger, sexual interest, and interpersonal frustration based on the in-session role plays. As he more frequently achieved his DOs and was able to recognize the role that his thoughts and behaviors played in attaining them, Sam was able to identify thoughts about his negative emotions that were hurtful in achieving his DOs ("I feel guilty for finding her attractive") and DOs that were impossible ("I wanted to not be angry"). The following section contains a sample CSQ from the first month of therapy and a form completed after several months of treatment.

Transcript 1

> *Step 1.* Describe what happened:
> > I was in my class when another student sat down near me, smiled, and waved. After class, I struck up a conversation with her. She declined to get together with me at the time but said we could study together closer to the next test date.

> *Step 2.* Describe your interpretations of what happened:
> > My beliefs create my reality, literally. I had to struggle against feelings of helplessness to a degree. I feel that part of me was holding myself back to a degree. I'm not sure what I'm supposed to learn from this situation. Whatever the outcome, it will reflect what is going on inside of me. Isolation is reflected by the outcome: I would have approached someone who would have accepted or someone who would have accepted would have sat next to me.

> *Step 3.* Describe what you did during the situation:
> > When she sat down near me, I noticed that she was not sitting in her normal seat. I began to check her out. When she smiled

and waved at me briefly, I noted her behavior as well and decided to approach her after class. During class, I felt a little anxious about my future course of action and turned my attention inward to grow more quiet inside. After class, I lingered briefly until I caught her attention. She asked if I had another class in the same room afterwards and I responded that I didn't. I asked her how she liked the class so far. I listened attentively to her answer, asked her more questions as she told me a little about herself, and responded to her questions. When she mentioned that she had a lot of studying to do for the class, I asked if she'd like to get together to study sometime. When she declined, saying that she was very busy right now, and described the things that were keeping her busy at the time and causing her some stress, I offered to get together with her sometime, if she ever wanted to unwind. When she said that she was too busy at the time but wouldn't mind getting together to study sometime closer to the test, I agreed. I offered to exchange numbers, but she said we could wait until closer to the test. We said goodbye, and I left.

Step 4. Describe how the event came out for you:
The interaction seemed somewhat positive, but no clear progress was made during the exchange in terms of creating further interaction in the future, which was disappointing.

Step 5. Describe how you wanted the event to come out for you:
I would have liked for the interaction to indicate mutual interest and attraction on both our parts and to have clearly demonstrated that further close interaction was likely.

Transcript 2 (several months into therapy)

Step 1. Describe what happened:
I called someone who responded to an e-mail I had sent, and we talked for awhile but didn't end up going out that night.

Step 2. Describe your interpretations of what happened:
I really want to go out with someone. I could set something up for later in the week. I'm a little nervous. I'm expecting trouble. I'm nervous and could choose to be calm to help me ask her out. Don't be timid. Be aware of my attitude so I don't self-defeat. I'm calm and pleasant. This is going okay so far. She can't go out tonight, but we can make plans for another time.

5. PERSONALITY DISORDER NOT OTHERWISE SPECIFIED

Step 3. Describe what you did during the situation:
I picked up the phone to call this woman after getting back from class. I hesitated with the phone in my hand for a few seconds because I had become a little nervous and scared at the thought of making the call. I reminded myself not to act timid and made the call. When she picked up, I said hello, asked how she was doing, and briefly talked about how I had just moved. We chatted about movies for a couple of minutes. I noticed that I didn't sound nervous, my voice sounded calm and at ease, but I noticed that we accidentally spoke at the same times a couple times I think because I was nervous on the inside. I asked her if she'd like to go out that night. She said she had plans.

Step 4. Describe how the event came out for you:
I tried to get together with someone that night, but it didn't work out.

Step 5. Describe how you wanted the event to come out for you:
I wanted to get together with someone that night.

Progress

Improvement was observed following several more months of practice using the CSQ and a willingness by Sam to make attempts at expressing his attraction or acknowledging his anger. Specifically, Sam learned that by acknowledging and expressing these emotions that he had labeled as negative, he reduced his anxiety during situations, was able to achieve his goals rather than thwart them, and felt less guilt and distress over situations in which his DO was not achieved.

After approximately 1 year of treatment, Sam's dysthymic symptoms were in remission, and many of his schizotypal and avoidant personality symptoms had improved. During the following 5 months, the CBASP treatment approach remained unchanged with the goal of ensuring maintenance of symptom reduction and increasing comfort with his new social skills and moderated philosophical beliefs. After 17 months of treatment, Sam requested that therapy be terminated. He felt that he had met his goals of reducing dysthymic symptoms and establishing a social network. Sam stated that he had learned the skills necessary to maintain his positive gains on his own.

Furthermore, with respect to the CSQ, he stated that he "did it automatically in his head" and no longer felt the need to complete the forms in therapy. At termination, Sam did not have diagnoses on Axes I, II, III or IV and his Global Assessment of Functioning rating was 85.

OBSTACLES TO TREATMENT

We have used CBASP to treat patients with PD NOS and have seen improvement in many personality symptoms. Despite these improvements, several difficulties often arose during the course of treatment and are likely to be encountered in other settings when treating these patients with various personality disorder features.

One of the earliest difficulties therapists are likely to encounter in using the CSQ is the intrinsic cognitions associated with personality disorders. Patients with personality disorders have dysfunctional beliefs that are entrenched in their cognitive organization and thus require significant time and effort to modify. Furthermore, many personality-disordered patients do not regard their personality traits as dysfunctional unless they are associated with other symptoms, such as depression or suicidal symptoms (Beck & Freeman, 1990).

Another difficulty in treating PD NOS is choosing thoughts and behaviors to prioritize with the CSQ. Whereas thoughts related to helplessness, hopelessness, and assertiveness are consistently chosen as matters of intervention for the treatment of patients with depressive disorders, it can often be unclear how to prioritize the thoughts and behaviors of PD NOS patients who present with symptoms of several personality disorders. As the treatment of these patients evolved in our clinic, it became evident that a clear conceptualization of the patient's personality symptoms was necessary to target the thoughts and behaviors that most severely impaired the patient. After determining which thoughts and behaviors to target, it is essential that therapists make it a priority because many patients have difficulty generating thoughts and behaviors to include in the CSQ, or they generate thoughts and behaviors that are unrelated to it.

A third difficulty in using the CSQ relates to the management of interpersonal difficulties between the therapist and patient, potentially inherent in any therapeutic relationship and particularly salient in personality-disordered patients. For example, with an individual with paranoid fea-

5. PERSONALITY DISORDER NOT OTHERWISE SPECIFIED

tures, it may be necessary to spend more time establishing a high level of trust before asking him or her to share, in minute detail, the specific content of thoughts and actions. Similarly, it is necessary for the therapist to resist the temptation to generate the entire content of the CSQ for an individual with dependent features. For an individual with schizotypal features, it is imperative that therapists be aware of the impact the patient is having on them, including frustration, confusion, or annoyance, and to use these feelings and thoughts as targets of intervention rather than allowing them to disengage the therapists.

A fourth potential obstacle in treating patients with PD NOS using the CSQ is the generation of alternative thoughts and behaviors that are both suitable to the patient and socially acceptable. By definition, the diagnosis of any personality disorder implies that an individual demonstrates an enduring, pervasive, and inflexible pattern of inner experience and behavior that deviates from norms. Due to the pervasiveness and rigidity of these symptoms, patients with personality disorders may be resistant to change and may feel sadness, confusion, or discomfort over the loss of beliefs and behaviors that have been so familiar. Consequently, the therapist must keep in mind that through the course of therapy, a patient is likely to undergo a type of role transition that is accompanied by fear, sadness, and adjustment to the new patterns of behavior. For example, in the case study presented previously, Sam, a patient with a diagnosis of PD NOS with schizotypal and avoidant features, was faced with challenging deeply ingrained philosophical beliefs on which he based much of his behavior. Acknowledging that some of the behaviors were interfering with his strong desire for social intimacy led to grief over the loss of his old beliefs and behaviors. Therefore, for patients with PD NOS, it is essential to manage grief or discomfort at the loss of certain patterns of behavior while encouraging the development of new skills that will help in achieving DOs.

The use of the CSQ treatment approach was successful with Sam. The information presented in this chapter is a case study, representing a mere beginning to consistent successful treatment of patients with PD NOS. This specific example, however, demonstrates that application of the CBASP technique may be useful in altering the deeply ingrained, persistent, maladaptive thoughts and behaviors present in personality-disordered patients. Furthermore, patients with PD NOS often present many interpersonal anomalies that make efficiency and consistency of treatment difficult to maintain, thereby decreasing treatments' effectiveness. The CBASP technique, however, may improve treatment efficiency in this group by providing a consistent structure and a predictable therapeutic agenda. Although future research is still needed to empirically validate the efficacy of the CBASP technique for patients with PD NOS, the initial findings in our clinic suggest that successful treatment and maintenance of treatment gains in these patients is indeed possible.

PART II

Anxiety Disorders

Chapter 6

Social Anxiety Disorder and Avoidant Personality Disorder*

This chapter demonstrates how the Cognitive Behavioral Analysis System of Psychotherapy can be easily incorporated, and in fact dovetails nicely, with existing empirically validated treatments for social anxiety disorder (e.g., exposure). Moreover, the incremental efficacy of integrating the present approach is depicted in the transcripts of actual therapy sessions with Fred, a 19-year-old with severe social anxiety and comorbid depressive symptoms. The Cognitive Behavioral Analysis System of Psychotherapy effectively targeted the specific behaviors and cognitions that contributed to Fred's long-term avoidance of social interactions, until his desired outcome of either endured or thwarted anxiety was regularly attained across a variety of interpersonal contexts. A discussion of common problems and difficulties in treating this pernicious, but treatable, condition is also provided.

As recently noted by Barlow, Raffa, and Cohen (2002), Social Anxiety Disorder (SAD) may be the most prevalent anxiety disorder (lifetime prevalence of 13%) and the third most prevalent of all mental disorders. According to the *Diagnostic and Statistical Manual of Mental Disorders–Fourth Edition* (*DSM–IV*; American Psychiatric Association, 1994), SAD has a typical onset in midadolescence with a continuous course and lifelong duration if untreated. It is more common in women than in men in community samples. SAD involves "a marked and persistent fear of one or more social or performance situations in which the person is exposed to unfamiliar people or to possible scrutiny by others" (American Psychiatric Associ-

---

*The primary authors contributing to this chapter were Bradley A. White, Kelly C. Cukrowicz, and Ginnette C. Blackhart.

ation, 1994, p. 416). Individuals with SAD also fear humiliation or embarrassment and usually experience anxiety and, sometimes, panic attacks upon exposure to feared social situations. Adults with SAD recognize that their fear is unreasonable or exaggerated. Nevertheless, they typically avoid or endure feared situations with intense anxious anticipation or distress, which interferes significantly with their normal functioning in social, academic, or occupational realms. In such individuals, this fear is not better attributed to medical conditions, substance abuse, or to other mental disorders (American Psychiatric Association, 1994). Frequently comorbid disorders include specific phobias, agoraphobia, generalized anxiety disorder, substance abuse, major depression, dysthymia, and obsessive-compulsive disorder (Schneier, Johnson, Hornig, Liebowitz, & Weissman, 1992).

SAD is specified as generalized if the fears include most social situations. In such cases, Avoidant Personality Disorder (APD) is considered as an additional diagnosis on Axis II. According to the *DSM–IV* (American Psychiatric Association, 1994, p. 664), APD is characterized by "a pervasive pattern of social inhibition, feelings of inadequacy, and hypersensitivity to negative evaluation, beginning by early adulthood and present in a variety of contexts." At least four features must be present, including avoidance of activities that could result in criticism, rejection, or disapproval; fear-based restraint in intimate relationships; preoccupation in social situations with criticism or rejection; inhibition in new social situations; a self-view as socially inept, inferior, or unappealing; and a reluctance to take risks or engage in new activities due to fear of embarrassment. Debate is ongoing regarding the relationship between SAD (particularly the generalized type) and APD and treatment outcome (e.g., Brown, Heimberg, & Juster, 1995). Herein, we regard generalized SAD and APD as essentially identical with regard to treatment implications. The interested reader is referred to other sources for information on the etiology of SAD (e.g., Barlow et al., 2002; Beck & Freeman, 1990; Hope & Heimberg, 1993; Schlenker & Leary, 1982).

EXISTING TREATMENTS FOR SAD AND APD

The most effective psychosocial treatment for SAD is combined exposure and cognitive behavioral therapy (CBT; Barlow et al., 2002). Barlow and colleagues suggest that exposure is the crucial element and that cognitive exercises enhance the effects of exposure. We concur and describe how the Cognitive Behavioral Analysis System of Psychotherapy (CBASP; McCullough, 2000) is a useful adjunct to exposure. Exposure involves repeated confrontation with the feared situation, in vivo with natural stimuli, via imaginal exercises, or through role plays, until habituation of the anxious response occurs (Barlow et al., 2002), whereas the cognitive aspect of traditional CBT emphasizes the identification, evaluation, and modification of logically distorted, anxiety-inducing thoughts. A group version of CBT for SAD (Cognitive Behavioral Group Therapy, or CBGT), described later, has also been shown to be effective (Hope & Heimberg, 1993).

Although social skills training and relaxation techniques (e.g., progressive muscle relaxation) have not been shown to on their own successfully treat SAD, they may be useful adjuncts when exposure and CBT are combined. Less research has been conducted on psychosocial interventions for the treatment of APD, although group-administered behavioral interventions involving exposure or social skills training have received some support (Crits-Christoph & Barber, 2002).

Several pharmacological treatments also exist for SAD, with selective serotonin reuptake inhibitors receiving the most scientific support and showing fewer side effects than monoamine oxidase inhibitors, tricyclic antidepressants, benzodiazapines, or beta blockers (Roy-Byrne & Cowley, 2002). However, there is little research on long-term efficacy of pharmacological interventions for SAD (Roy-Byrne & Cowley, 2002), and there are no controlled studies of pharmacotherapy specifically for APD (Koenigsberg, Woo-Ming, & Siever, 2002). Pharmacological and psychosocial interventions such as CBASP are not necessarily mutually exclusive and can even work synergistically (Keller et al., 2000). However, questions remain as to whether antianxiety medications interfere with psychosocial interventions for SAD, and Hope and Heimberg (1993) recommend that patients reduce or at least stabilize intake of antianxiety medications under a physician's supervision before undertaking CBGT. We recommend that therapists stay abreast of patients' medications and air concerns while deferring to prescribers as arbiters of change to medication regimens.

CBASP AS A SEPARATE OR SUPPLEMENTAL TREATMENT

Although our propositions must await empirical validation, there are a number of reasons to anticipate incremental efficacy and use of integrating the principles and procedures of CBASP with established psychosocial and pharmacological treatments of SAD and APD. First, CBASP has recently been shown to be a highly efficacious form of cognitive behavioral therapy for treatment-resistant chronic depression, particularly when combined with pharmacotherapy (Keller et al., 2000). Second, the high comorbidity of anxiety and depression suggests that these disorders may share common etiological mechanisms, and they seem to be similarly responsive to particular interventions (CBT and behavioral activation/exposure). Third, CBASP's emphasis on evaluating interpretations based on personal goals (functionality vs. veridicality, per traditional CBT) seems particularly likely to help patients with SAD and APD to reduce self-criticism and develop greater self-determination (Ryan & Deci, 2000). Fourth, socially anxious individuals tend to underestimate successes and thereby miss valuable positive experiences. Using CBASP to examine success situations in which Desired Outcomes (DOs) are achieved can further stimulate self-efficacy beliefs and motivation. Fifth, socially anxious individuals tend to unproductively focus or shift attention in a biased or unsystematic fashion, further exacerbating anxious arousal. Mastery of CBASP helps replace this habit with a more productive, systematic, problem-solving approach. Finally, CBASP emphasizes social problems and interpersonal relationships, the primary realms affected in SAD and APD.

APPLYING CBASP TO THE TREATMENT OF SAD AND APD

The fundamental techniques of McCullough's (2000) CBASP for chronic depression are applicable to patients with SAD and APD, and the general format for the Coping Survey Questionnaire (CSQ) elicitation and remediation phases is the same. However, certain modifications and applications of CBASP appear to enhance intervention for SAD and APD. For the sake of chapter organization, we consider both elicitation and remediation phases in the same section for each step of the CSQ. However, it is imperative to teach patients to systematically complete the full elicitation phase of each CSQ prior to beginning the remediation phase, following traditional CBASP.

Preliminary Interventions

The elaboration and remediation of CSQs requires focused concentration, particularly before the technique has become automatic. Anxious arousal interferes with concentration, and patients with SAD and APD may have difficulty focusing on CSQ work when they are experiencing anxious arousal invoked by the therapist's presence, the recall of distressing situ-

6. SOCIAL ANXIETY AND AVOIDANT PERSONALITY DISORDERS

ations, or generalized worry. Therefore, we sometimes find it helpful to teach patients to practice standard relaxation exercises (e.g., breathing, imagery, or progressive muscle relaxation) that they can employ to regulate their emotional state and achieve a mindset conducive to completing CSQs.

Situations

The first step of the elicitation phase of the CSQ requires the patient to describe a temporally discrete, specific situation. Performance evaluation and interpersonal situations are usually the most distressing to individuals with SAD and APD, and thus they are among the best candidates for use with the CSQ in the treatment of these disorders. Such situations include, but are not limited to, public speaking or performing, initiating and engaging in conversations, dating, interacting with authority figures, attending parties or social events, using public restrooms, writing or eating in public, exercising or playing sports, interviewing, shopping, being assertive or expressing opinions, and dealing with conflicts. Such situations are also useful to consider in patients' construction of fear hierarchies and exposure assignments, which are described later.

Patients with SAD and APD tend to underestimate and underreport the frequency of positive social experiences and to discount their influence in success situations, in which anxiety was thwarted or endured so that DOs were attained. It is important to train socially anxious patients to be on the lookout for, and to complete CSQs, for success situations as well as for situations in which DOs were not attained. Doing so helps patients recognize therapeutic gains, overcome the habit of discounting the positive, and identify interpretations and behaviors that helped them achieve their DOs and manage their anxiety.

Due to extensive avoidance, patients with generalized SAD and APD often have infrequent or restricted experience with natural social situations. With such patients, CSQs may initially focus almost exclusively on in-session role plays and in vivo exposure homework assignments, while patients work to find ways to increase the frequency of natural social encounters.

Situational Interpretations

In the second step of the elicitation phase of the CSQ, patients identify several interpretations of the situation at the time it occurred. When asking the patient what the event meant to him or her, it can be helpful for the therapist to be aware of the general interpretation patterns of socially anxious individuals. Individuals with SAD and APD are frequently perfectionistic, pessimistic, hypervigilant for threat cues, hypersensitive to criticism and rejection, dependent, self-deprecating, and low in self-esteem, distress tolerance, and acceptance of self and others. They may make global judgments of self-worth based on performance. They are also prone to many of the cognitive distortions that are labeled in traditional CBT, including fortune telling, mind reading, all-or-nothing thinking, personalization, overgeneralization, magnification and minimization, arbitrary inference, catastrophic and probabilistic thinking, and underestimation of social skills. McCullough (2000, Table 6.3, p.122) and Beck and Freeman (1990) provide excellent reviews of additional cognitive themes relevant to patients with SAD and APD that can affect attainment of DOs.

During the remediation phase, patients evaluate and revise irrelevant and inaccurate interpretations based primarily on the main criterion—"Did this interpretation help or hurt the attainment of my desired outcome?" Patients may also evaluate interpretations with regard to the following questions: "Was this relevant?" and "Did it reflect what was actually happening in this situation?"

Additional Step: Subjective Units of Distress Scale

When using CSQs in the treatment of SAD, it can be useful to also elicit from patients the subjective level of anxiety corresponding with each interpretation as it occurred. This addition helps patients see the link between thoughts and emotions, and it provides a simple way to quantify and monitor progress in reducing anxiety symptoms. A convenient measure for this purpose is the Subjective Units of Distress Scale (SUDS) ratings (Wolpe & Lazarus, 1966), used regularly in CBGT. Patients assign a numerical value to their anxiety on a 100-point scale that has reference points at 25 (*mild anxiety*), 50 (*moderate; beginning to have difficulty concentrating*), 75 (*high; thoughts of escaping*), and 100 points (*worst anxiety ever experienced or imaginable*). As in CBGT, patients can be trained to give SUDS ratings at various intervals during in-session exposures as well, as discussed later.

Situational Behavior

In the next step of the elicitation phase, patients are asked to describe their behaviors in the situation, including both what they did and how they did it (e.g., tone and volume of voice, posture, mannerisms, facial expressions).

6. SOCIAL ANXIETY AND AVOIDANT PERSONALITY DISORDERS   87

The most common problematic behaviors associated with SAD and APD are partial or complete avoidance, escape, and safety behaviors; unassertive or passive-aggressive actions; excessive reassurance seeking; social skill implementation deficits; and substance use. These behaviors may be very subtle, sophisticated, and automatic, occurring outside the patients' awareness. The therapist should watch for undisclosed details and have patients reenact their situational behavior in session whenever necessary. Common examples of goal-interfering behavior include being mentally distracted (including worrying over task-irrelevant matters), procrastinating, busying oneself with work, overpreparing or rehearsing, reading or wearing headphones, always attending events with a friend, or hiding signs of anxiety (blushing, avoiding eye contact) with makeup, hair, clothing, or sunglasses.

In the remediation phase, the patient determines whether behaviors must be replaced or added to increase the odds of attaining the DO. Socially anxious patients often have at least a good conceptual grasp of, if not practice with, helpful behaviors, although they may fear the potential consequences of trying out these behaviors in a new situation. At other times, however, there exists a true skill or implementation deficit, particularly in patients with generalized SAD and APD, whose social skill repertoire may be underdeveloped across social settings due to extensive avoidance. In either instance, after verbal remediation of behaviors on the CSQ, it can be very helpful to have the patient rehearse desirable behaviors via role play, with the therapist modeling appropriate behaviors first if necessary. Therapists should illuminate distinctions between passive (other's needs over one's own), assertive (both own and other's needs considered) and aggressive (own needs over other's) behavior because socially anxious patients often confuse passivity with being nice and assertiveness with being aggressive or mean.

Desired Outcomes

The next and arguably most important step in CSASP involves clearly specifying the DO in the situation. When asking socially anxious people how they want the situation to come out, it is crucial that the patient identify and select only one DO and state it in objective, specific, observable terms. To ensure that the latter requirements are met, the therapist can ask, "How would an observer know that you had attained your desired outcome? What would he or she see?"

In traditional CBASP, patients are asked to specify a single DO at the time of the situation. However, patients with SAD and APD sometimes generate DOs that reduce anxiety in the short term, via escape or avoidance, but conflict with long-term objectives, such as becoming more comfortable in similar situations over time or learning to endure some discomfort to pursue personal goals. Because only one DO can be attained for any situation, SAD or APD patients must learn to prioritize long-term DOs over potentially conflicting short-term goals, such as always making favorable impressions, winning social approval, performing perfectly, or immediately reducing or hiding anxiety symptoms. The therapist can support the patient in this endeavor by maintaining a nonconfrontational approach and empathizing with the patient's immediate goals, while encouraging the patient to consider his or her long-term goals to ensure that these are being served by the DO the patient generated. As McCullough (2000) noted, patients typically come to recognize on their own the unattainability of unrealistic or conflicting DOs after repeated practice with CSQs. On the other hand, we find that it is beneficial to explain to patients (and subsequently elicit from them through examples) the benefits of tolerating the short-term discomfort of exposure to anxiety-invoking situations for the sake of long-term personal goals, including increased comfort in social situations.

Actual Outcomes

In the last step of the CSQ elicitation phase, patients generate a single, observable Actual Outcome (AO) for the situation that is anchored in time and stated in objective behavioral terms, rather than ambiguous or emotional terms (although it can be acknowledged verbally or with additional SUDS ratings that feelings usually accompany objective outcomes). Deleterious consequences of avoidant or unassertive behaviors should be explored if the patient is not forthcoming, for instance, by asking "What else came out of this situation?" Patients are then asked to compare the AO to the DO to determine whether the DO was achieved.

Application of DOs to Exposure
and Anxiety-Reduction Goals

Another potential modification to the traditional use of CBASP in the treatment of SAD and APD is the application of CSQs to plan for and monitor exposure assignments. Habituation and long-term anxiety reduction is most effective when the individual remains in the exposure situations long enough to notice a reduction in their anxiety. Exposure assign-

6. SOCIAL ANXIETY AND AVOIDANT PERSONALITY DISORDERS 89

ments are typically based on a fear hierarchy list created by the patient, starting with exposure to situations that are identified as causing only slight discomfort and gradually progressing over time toward situations at the top of the hierarchy (i.e., those that cause tremendous discomfort). Regular SUDS ratings can help the therapist and patient monitor for sufficient habituation in both simulated and in vivo exposure situations.

It may at times be desirable for the patient to define DOs in terms of remaining in the exposure situation until he or she reaches a target SUDS level. However, it is very important that the DO focus on behavioral elements, such as staying in the exposure situation, perhaps for a predetermined minimum amount of time (e.g., 20 min), rather than vaguely defining the DO as the attainment of a particular SUDS level or feeling, such as "not being anxious." Consistent with the traditional CBT model, we view emotional change (including anxiety reduction) as the product of changes in interpretations and behavior. Overfocusing attention and effort on the immediate control or reduction of anxious feelings is not only misdirected, but also it can have the paradoxical effect of increasing one's distress, to which many patients with social anxiety can attest. Instead, we favor DOs that emphasize a proactive approach toward one's personal goals despite anxiety, while allowing oneself to experience in an accepting, nonjudgmental fashion whatever feelings one is having at the time. This view is consistent with modern mindfulness/acceptance-based approaches to CBT for other disorders, including Generalized Anxiety Disorder, which often coincides with SAD and APD (e.g., Linehan, 1993a; Roemer & Orsillo, 2002). As patients may confuse acceptance with giving up attempts to change, it can be helpful to clarify distinctions between demanding/catastrophic, accepting/tolerant, and resigned/acquiescent stances. Albert Ellis' (2001) rational emotive approach of rewording "should" and "must" interpretations (e.g., "I should/must not feel anxious") as "like" and "prefer" statements (e.g., "I would like/prefer to feel less anxious") is highly consistent with and appropriate for acceptance-oriented CSQ interpretation remediation for patients with SAD and APD.

Comparing AOs and DOs and Remediation

McCullough's (2000) CBASP remediation phase is largely unmodified for the treatment of SAD and APD. Patients are asked, "Did you get what you wanted in this situation?" Although the answer to this question may appear self-evident, having patients explicitly acknowledge it crucially illuminates the match or discrepancy between AO and DO, as well as the patients' responsibility for attainment of their personal goals, motivating them toward change.

During the remediation phase, patients are asked to examine each interpretation in terms of relevancy to the situation, accuracy, and, especially, whether and how it helped or impeded the patient in obtaining the DO. The same procedure is repeated next with each situational behavior. If an unattainable or unrealistic DO is identified along the way, the patient is asked to revise it according to the guidelines described earlier before proceeding. Although it can be very tempting to answer remediation questions for the patient or argue with their responses, doing so defeats the collaborative and agency-promoting benefits of the CBASP approach.

After labeling each interpretation and behavior as helpful or hurtful, patients revise or add interpretations and behaviors to increase the likelihood of attaining the DO. If social skills deficits are identified, the patient can be guided toward several potential alternative behaviors, asked how these might affect the likelihood of achieving the DO, and encouraged to rehearse selected behaviors following the therapist's lead. After the remediation phase is completed, it can also be worthwhile to briefly discuss general patterns (e.g., "How does this pattern apply to similar situations you've experienced?").

Application of CBASP to CBGT

In addition to its application to individual treatment, we found that CBASP is easily modified for use in conjunction with CBGT for SAD, developed by Hope and Heimberg (1993). This empirically supported treatment involves in-session exposure exercises, traditional cognitive restructuring exercises, and progressive in vivo exposure assignments administered in a group format. At the Florida State University Psychology Clinic, we have begun to integrate CBASP with CBGT to enhance patient motivation and acceptance. In addition to group sessions, members typically attend weekly individual therapy sessions, in which they learn the fundamentals of CBASP (illustrated later in our case example). In group sessions, patients are asked to identify their DOs for in-session role plays and in vivo homework situations and to articulate how modifying distorted cognitions and behaviors will help them to achieve their DOs. We have observed anecdotally that having our CBGT patients consider the impact of their interpretations on DO attainment enhances their

6. SOCIAL ANXIETY AND AVOIDANT PERSONALITY DISORDERS

acceptance, mindfulness, and self-determination in anxiety-invoking situations.

⟶ CASE EXAMPLE ⟵

To illustrate how CBASP can be incorporated into CBT for SAD and APD, we present a case study of an adult in therapy for SAD and APD at the Florida State University Psychology Clinic.

Fred was a 19-year-old college student beginning his sophomore year when he came to the clinic seeking treatment for SAD. Fred's social anxiety inhibited his life in a number of ways. Although he was able to participate in most solitary and family activities, he reported experiencing a great deal of anxiety in all situations in which he would have to be around or interact with others. This included walking on campus, being in class, going to the mall, going to the grocery store, eating in restaurants, going to the movies, talking on the telephone, having to speak in class, going to parties, and having to talk to others (individuals or groups). He was bothered by autonomic arousal symptoms (e.g., sweaty palms, racing heart) and constantly worried about what others might be thinking or saying about him, believing that they were negatively evaluating him. He was unable to make eye contact with others or to initiate or maintain conversations with other people.

Fred reported that he had experienced some social anxiety since the age of 12 but that it had become much more severe since beginning college. He had no friends or acquaintances, and he had never been on a date. His family was his only source of social support, and, although he was extremely close to them, they lived several hours away. Fred reported experiencing quite a bit of loneliness as well as some depressive symptoms, including occasional suicidal thoughts. Fred was diagnosed with SAD, Generalized Type, and APD. He was also diagnosed with Depressive Disorder Not Otherwise Specified because his aforementioned depression symptoms did not meet criteria for Major Depressive Disorder.

FRED'S TREATMENT PLAN

The treatment plan for Fred consisted of CBT for Social Phobia based on Leahy and Holland (2000), including relaxation training, exposure to feared situations, and cognitive restructuring. CBASP techniques were also incorporated into treatment using the CSQ. During the first two therapy sessions, Fred was taught progressive muscle relaxation and deep-breathing exercises as ways to manage his feelings of anxiety when in social situations and to reduce anxious arousal when necessary before completing CSQs. A fear hierarchy was also developed and implemented in exposure using SUDS ratings. The rationale of the CSQ and how to use it in conjunction with the exposure assignments were discussed with Fred.

Because Fred initially presented with comorbid depression and suicidal ideation, the therapist chose to address these symptoms using traditional CBASP alone during the first several weeks of therapy, without additional exposure assignments. Fred quickly mastered the CSQ framework, and his depressive symptoms decreased substantially over this time. Next, in-session role plays and in vivo exposure assignments were gradually integrated into the treatment based on Fred's hierarchy. After attempting an exposure assignment, Fred completed a CSQ on the exposure situation.

The following is a vignette (abbreviated to focus on just one interpretation and one behavior) of Fred and his therapist discussing a CSQ in session near the beginning of therapy on an exposure assignment Fred completed. The therapist began with the elicitation phase.

Therapist: Let's look at the CSQ. Here the assignment was that you were to make eye contact with someone and greet that person.

Fred: Yeah. I went to the grocery store Friday night, and when I was going through the checkout line, I said hello to the grocery clerk and asked her how she was doing.

Therapist: Okay, now on to Step 2. What were your interpretations or thoughts when you were in that situation?

Fred: One of my thoughts was "I'm not normal because I am here alone."

Therapist: Okay. So one of your interpretations in this situation was "I'm not normal because I am here alone." I see your SUDS rating for this thought was 90. This seems to be a good interpretation for us to focus on. Now let's move on to Step 3. What were your behaviors in that situation?

Fred: While I was in the grocery store, I kept my head down the entire time and looked at the floor or nothing at all, except when I looked at the clerk and made eye contact with her.

6. SOCIAL ANXIETY AND AVOIDANT PERSONALITY DISORDERS 93

Therapist: What else did you do?

Fred: I just pretty much kept my head down and did not talk to anyone, except for when I asked the clerk how she was doing. So I said, "Hi," and asked her how she was doing but said it very softly.

Therapist: Did the clerk respond?

Fred: Yes, she said she was doing fine. But then I couldn't think of anything else to say, so I looked back down and didn't say anything else.

Therapist: So your behaviors in this situation were to keep your head down and look at the floor and not to talk to anyone, except when you greeted the clerk.

Fred: Yes.

Therapist: Let's move on to Step 4. What was your DO?

Fred: To go to the grocery store and get my groceries without any stress.

Therapist: And what was the AO?

Fred: I got my groceries, but my SUDS was about 85 or 90. I was able to make eye contact with the grocery clerk and ask her how she was doing.

Therapist: Did you achieve your DO, then?

Fred: Sort of. I was able to make eye contact with the clerk and speak to her, but I wasn't able to talk to anyone else or even look at anyone else, and I still experienced a lot of stress.

Therapist: It sounds like you may have actually had two DOs, then. One was to get your groceries without experiencing any stress. But it also seems like another DO for you was to be to make eye contact and greet a person while in the grocery store. Do you think that is true?

Fred: I guess so. I was able to look at the clerk and ask her how she was doing. But I still experienced a lot of anxiety while in the grocery store, and I couldn't think of anything else to say to the woman at the checkout counter.

Fred initially described more than one DO that included both short-term and long-term goals: to go to the grocery store and to make eye contact with someone and greet that person (his AO) as well as to keep the conversation going and not experience any distress (goals he did not attain). The therapist therefore asked Fred whether going to the grocery store and not experiencing any stress was a realistic DO, and Fred agreed that it was not. He then formulated a compromise between his goals and revised his DO to state "Make eye contact with someone, say 'hello,' and ask the person how he or she is doing [thereby completing his exposure assignment], while attempting to accept and tolerate feelings of anxiety." The transcript continues following this revision.

Therapist: So did you get this corrected DO?

Fred: I suppose so. But I still wasn't able to think of anything else to say, and my SUDS level was about 90 when I spoke to the grocery clerk, which bothered me a lot.

After acknowledging that he actually only partially attained his DO, Fred and his therapist moved on to the remediation phase:

Therapist: Okay, then, let's go back through your interpretations to see which ones were helpful and hurtful to you in getting your DO of making eye contact with someone and greeting the person, while tolerating any anxiety. Your first interpretation was, "I am not normal because I am here alone." Do you think that thought was helpful or hurtful to you in this situation?

Fred: Hurtful.

Therapist: Why?

Fred: Because I kept my head down and didn't speak to anyone because they would look at me and think I was weird because I was alone and because I was talking to them.

Therapist: Can you think of any thoughts, then, that you could replace the hurtful thought with that would be helpful to you in this situation?

Fred: I am normal.

Therapist: Good. How do you think that would have helped you?

Fred: Well, if I kept telling myself that I was normal and was not weird for being there alone, and that it's okay to feel anxious, I may have been more likely to have kept my head up and made eye contact with someone. I probably would have been more likely to say hello to someone.

Therapist: So telling yourself "I am normal and I am not weird for being here alone or feeling anxious" would have made it easier for you to keep your head up, make eye contact with others, and to talk to other people?

Fred: Yes.

Therapist: It seems, though, that in this situation you were able to do that. You made eye contact with the checkout clerk and greeted her.

6. SOCIAL ANXIETY AND AVOIDANT PERSONALITY DISORDERS 95

Fred: But I still felt a lot of anxiety, which really bothered me, and that made it harder to look up.

Therapist: Do you think that your replacement thought would have made you feel less anxious, then, or help you accept the anxiety you felt?

Fred: Probably. It would have been a lot easier for me.

Therapist: So your interpretation "I am not normal because I am here alone" was hurtful to you because it made you keep your head down and not speak to anyone while you were in the grocery store, except when you spoke to the clerk, and then you still experienced a lot of anxiety, which made you feel more uncomfortable. If you replaced that interpretation, then, with "I am normal and I am not weird for being here alone, and it's okay to feel anxious" you would have experienced less anxiety or been more accepting of it, and you would have been more likely to keep your head up and speak to others. Is that right?

Fred: Yes.

Therapist: Then let's move on to Step 3. One of your behaviors in this situation was to keep your head down the entire time, except when you made eye contact with the clerk. Do you think this was helpful or hurtful to you in achieving your DO?

Fred: Hurtful. I probably would have been more likely to make eye contact with other people and maybe even say hi if I didn't look down the entire time.

Therapist: But you were able to make eye contact and speak to the clerk. How was it hurtful, then?

Fred: While I was looking at the ground, I just kept thinking about how I wasn't normal and that I just wanted to leave.

Therapist: So keeping your head down actually made you think more negatively?

Fred: Yes. If I had my head up and looked at other people, I might have been distracted and not thought those things over and over again.

Therapist: Then, what behavior would have been helpful to you in this situation?

Fred: To keep my head up. I probably wouldn't have thought negatively as much and would have been more likely to make eye contact with others and to even speak to people in the grocery store.

Therapist: So in this situation, if you would have thought to yourself "I am normal and I am not weird for being here alone, and it's okay to feel anxiety" instead of, "I am not normal because I am here

> alone, and I shouldn't feel anxiety," and if you would have kept your head up instead of looking at the ground the entire time, you would have been more likely to get your entire DO, which was to make eye contact and greet someone while feeling less anxiety and better tolerating the anxiety you did feel, right?
>
> *Fred:* Yes.

During the elicitation phase, Fred identified several thoughts and behaviors that not only coincided to increase his anxiety in this social situation but also made it less likely that he would attain his DO. Fred also discovered that part of his initial DO was unrealistic and unattainable and partially conflicted with his long-term goals. The therapist thus asked Fred to immediately revise his DO before proceeding with the CSQ. During the remediation phase, Fred was able to generate plausible alternative interpretations and actions that he felt would increase the chance of attaining his revised DO.

Outcome

Fred's initial level of social anxiety and avoidance were quite painful and debilitating. After several months of individual and group therapy, Fred experienced dramatic improvement. He was able to master the CBASP method after six sessions and can complete the CSQ both after situations and prospectively. Fred continues to experience anxiety in social situations; however, his anxiety level has decreased substantially. During a recent exchange with a stranger, he reported an initial SUDS of 60 that decreased to 25 after 15 min of conversation. Fred was able to make eye contact, maintain his part of the conversation, laugh and smile, and ask this person to join him for a movie in the coming weeks. During the time Fred has been in therapy, he has attained employment, established relationships with several co-workers, given speeches in front of large groups of people, and played his guitar and sung in front of small groups. Fred continues to fear some social situations and experience anxiety while participating in them, but the level of anxiety and fear has decreased from a level that previously impaired his performance to a milder one. Fred is able to generate situational interpretations that are more likely to decrease his anxiety or help him accept and endure it (e.g., "I may be anxious, but I know I can do this"). He has also acquired social skills that make

6. SOCIAL ANXIETY AND AVOIDANT PERSONALITY DISORDERS   97

it less obvious that he is anxious in these situations (e.g., he maintains eye contact, smiles, and shows reduced extraneous bodily movement). Fred has also improved in his avoidance of feared situations. To date he has completed his initial hierarchy of feared situations and has established a second one consisting of exposure situations he felt were completely unrealistic at intake (e.g., talking to a woman and asking for a date). Fred has also improved significantly in his ability to carry out previously difficult daily tasks. Fred's depressive symptoms and suicidal ideation have fluctuated during therapy, but overall they have decreased significantly throughout the course of treatment.

OBSTACLES TO TREATMENT

A variety of obstacles may occur when implementing CBASP for SAD and APD. In addition to the challenges in completing the CSQ (addressed in previous chapters), obstacles specific to socially anxious patients often include the completion of exposure assignments, as well as general patient and therapeutic alliance factors discussed later. A first step in dealing with these challenges is to examine and resolve with the patient any problems in the therapeutic alliance (does the patient believe that the therapist adequately met him or her at point A before working to accompany him or her to B?). Second, it can be helpful to revisit regularly the rationale behind the treatment to maintain the patient's motivation to complete exposure and CSQ assignments despite distress and anxiety, while learning to accept such short-term fluctuations in comfort level. Additionally, exploring the patient's personal experience with anxiety by constructing a fear hierarchy also elucidates important issues to address through role plays, cognitive restructuring, and CBASP principles.

Obstacles to completing exposure assignments may manifest in various forms; however, in socially anxious patients, they most often originate from the apprehension and ambivalence SAD and APD patients feel about the challenges they must confront to experience positive change. For instance, patients may have low confidence in the likelihood of a positive outcome or in their ability to endure the situation. They may have real or perceived skills deficits that impede their performance, or they may fear negative evaluation by others. They may have failed in a previous situation similar to this exposure assignment, or they may believe that they cannot be assertive enough to complete the assignment. They may believe they cannot tolerate a high level of anxiety and that somehow their anxiety will eventually diminish without having to endure exposure.

A variety of procedures may be effective in addressing and rolling with resistance to the completion of exposure assignments; techniques of motivational interviewing (Miller & Rollnick, 2002) are helpful in this regard. Although avoidance behaviors may at times seem frustratingly irrational to the therapist, it is important to identify and address the function behind the patients' resistance and their beliefs that lead them to fail in completing assignments. As described earlier, the therapist should help find and validate the kernel of truth in these concerns, acknowledging the pros and cons of continued avoidance, while asking the patient whether the long-term advantages of confrontation outweigh the short-term disadvantages, in light of his or her DOs. The therapist can also have patients explain their understanding of the rationale for completing exposure assignments. Another strategy is to highlight previous successes for the patient, including situations in which the patient was initially resistant to but ultimately succeeded in confronting and handling the exposure. The therapist can ask the patient to identify parallels between interpretations in the previous situation and the current one. When a patient is particularly sure that he or she "just can't do it," it can help to role play the situation in session, with the therapist first modeling the role of the patient. Once this role play is complete, the therapist can congratulate the patient on his or her courage and effort and ask the patient to identify several positive aspects of his or her own performance (without disqualifying the positive). The patient's fear hierarchy is also useful for monitoring and highlighting progress, while balancing the push for change with acceptance for the patient's current level of functioning and personal goals for therapy.

Individual patient factors can create obstacles in treatment for SAD and APD with CBASP. These may include suicidality, therapy-interfering behavioral patterns, trust issues, comorbidity, and acceptance issues. Each therapist delivering this treatment needs to assess these factors carefully to determine the impact they might have on the treatment implementation. The most important of these factors is suicidality. This should be assessed thoroughly during every session for a patient that presents with suicidal ideation (see Joiner, Walker, Rudd, & Jobes, 1999, for details of suicide assessment). After determining the impact these factors will have on therapy, the therapist should address them specifically with the patient and arrive at an agreement as to how they will be dealt with.

6. SOCIAL ANXIETY AND AVOIDANT PERSONALITY DISORDERS

Problems with therapeutic alliance can interfere with CBASP for SAD and APD. Patients must be able to trust that the therapist is not only knowledgeable and able to help but also concerned about them and their welfare. Beck and Freeman (1990) emphasize how the dysfunctional schemas of individuals with APD frequently manifest in the therapeutic relationship itself, reducing trust, compromising the therapeutic alliance, and retarding progress in treatment. As Beck and colleagues note, patients may not volunteer these cognitions even when they notice them. The therapist must communicate warmth, concern, validation, empathy, and respect toward patients, consider mindful self-disclosure (based on patients' needs), and nondefensively acknowledge and apologize for mistakes. Although the collaborative and acceptance-promoting nature of CBASP goes a long way to reduce alliance disturbances, we have found it to be extremely valuable to regularly elicit patients' current thoughts about the therapeutic process. Borrowing from Dialectic Behavioral Therapy techniques (Linehan, 1993a, 1993b), the therapist can elicit agreement from the patient early in therapy on the importance of developing a trusting relationship for therapy to work and a policy of openly discussing anything the therapist does that is bothersome to the patient.

Previous studies indicate that CBASP is an efficacious treatment for patients with chronic depression or dysthymia (Keller et al., 2000). This chapter focused on applying this treatment for patients with SAD or APD by combining CBASP with existing treatment modalities. This approach addresses a number of goals for patients with SAD and APD. It includes components of exposure, cognitive restructuring, and goal-oriented evaluation of previous situations as well as future situations. The mechanism of change with this therapeutic approach appears to rest on patients' mastery of the process of generating goal-oriented interpretations and behaviors. This approach seems likely to promote a sustained reduction in the symptoms of SAD and APD, as well as a variety of comorbid disorders. Although the efficacy of this treatment modality awaits further investigation, our experience with this application of CBASP to SAD and APD suggests that it is a simple and highly beneficial approach to intervention for these complex and disabling disorders.

Chapter 7

Generalized Anxiety Disorder and Panic Disorder*

Little modification of the Cognitive Behavioral Analysis System of Psychotherapy approach is actually needed to effectively target the maladaptive cognitions and behaviors thought to maintain both Panic Disorder and Generalized Anxiety Disorder. This chapter summarizes existing empirically validated treatments for Panic Disorder and Generalized Anxiety Disorder, but demonstrates that emphasis the Cognitive Behavioral Analysis System of Psychotherapy places on specific situations offers a practical advantage as an in-session means to manage the often diffuse, unfocused anxiety symptoms associated with each of these conditions. Two case descriptions illustrate the successful implementation of the system in the treatment of Panic Disorder and Generalized Anxiety Disorder in our outpatient clinic.

This chapter provides an overview of the application of McCullough's (2000) Cognitive Behavioral Analysis System of Psychotherapy (CBASP) and its structured component, the Coping Survey Questionnaire (CSQ), to anxiety disorders. Specifically, we discuss the value of integrating CBASP into empirically validated treatments for Panic Disorder (PD) and Generalized Anxiety Disorder (GAD). We offer specific recommendations for its application to treating these disorders and discuss some potential obstacles the therapist may encounter when applying CBASP and the CSQ to the treatments for PD and GAD.

---

*The primary authors contributing to this chapter were Ginette C. Blackhart and Sheila Stanley.

One of the most important components in the treatment of anxiety disorders is exposure, a behavioral technique emphasizing that one's anxiety only dissipates if one is exposed to the feared object or situation. Another important component of treatment for anxiety disorders is cognitive therapy, primarily because persons with anxiety disorders often experience cognitive distortions and worries. Therefore, by incorporating cognitive therapy into behavioral treatment for many anxiety disorders—including PD and GAD—the therapist not only exposes the patient to the feared object or situation but also targets the patient's worries and negative distorted cognitions.

Worry and cognitive distortions play a particularly important role in both PD and GAD. Those with PD (with or without Agoraphobia) often have catastrophic cognitions, which are inaccurate interpretations of the physical sensations they experience just before and during a panic attack (Zuckerman, 1999). In addition, they may constantly worry about experiencing future panic attacks and the consequences of the panic attacks (Barlow, Esler, & Vitali, 1998). Those with Agoraphobia (whether or not they are diagnosed with PD) constantly experience anxiety and worry about experiencing a panic attack or paniclike symptoms while in a public place, such as a shopping mall, restaurant, and so on. Finally, those with GAD experience constant worry that is mostly negative in content and difficult to control (American Psychiatric Association, 1994).

TREATMENTS FOR ANXIETY DISORDERS: WHAT CBASP HAS TO OFFER

Cognitive distortions and worry are key features in these anxiety disorders, and many empirical studies found that a combinination of cognitive therapy and behavioral treatments for PD, Agoraphobia, and GAD is more effective than behavioral treatments alone. Due to the cognitive component present in these anxiety disorders, and that the most successful treatments for these anxiety disorders include behavioral (i.e., exposure, relaxation) and cognitive components (Nathan & Gorman, 1998), it seems logical that the CSQ, used by McCullough (2000) in the treatment of depression, would be ideal for use with existing empirically validated treatments for these disorders. The CSQ (as explained in Chapter 1 and other chapters in this volume) encourages the patient to recognize his or her own interpretations (or cognitions) and behaviors in specific situations. These interpretations and behaviors are then evaluated and reanalyzed in terms of the outcome the patient desires in that specific situation (the Desired Outcome, or DO).

If empirically validated cognitive behavioral treatments for panic and GAD already exist (Barlow et al., 1998; Borkovec & Costello, 1993; Butler, Fennell, Robson, & Gelder, 1991), then why would the therapist want to incorporate CBASP into the treatment of these anxiety disorders? The answer is simple. CBASP is particularly useful in the treatment of anxiety disorders because it focuses the patient on his or her specific goals within a situation and on the goals of treatment, a task that can be difficult for patients with these anxiety disorders. As a supplement to the empirically validated treatments for PD and GAD, CBASP maintains the patient's attention on the specific goals of therapy, thereby increasing the likelihood that the patient will engage in exposure exercises and alter his or her cognitions and behaviors appropriately.

In the sections that follow, we show how CBASP may be specifically applied to the treatments for PD (with or without Agoraphobia) and GAD. Each section provides a detailed description of the symptoms of each disorder and their established empirically validated treatments, as well as any obstacles that may impede CBASP's implementation. Case examples are provided to better illustrate the use of CBASP as applied in our clinic.

CBASP APPLICATION TO PANIC DISORDER

The *Diagnostic and Statistical Manual of Mental Disorders* (*DSM–IV*; American Psychiatric Association, 1994) characterizes PD by the following criteria: recurrent, unexpected panic attacks and at least one of the attacks is followed by 1 month or more of persistent concern about having additional attacks, worry about the implications of the attack or its consequences, a significant change in behavior related to the attacks, or a combination of these criteria. A panic attack is defined as a discrete period of intense fear or discomfort, in which panic symptoms develop abruptly and reach a peak within 10 min. Four of the following symptoms must be present for this diagnosis:

1. Heart palpitations, pounding heart, or accelerated heart rate
2. Sweating, trembling, or shaking; shortness of breath
3. Feelings of choking; chest pain or discomfort
4. Nausea or abdominal distress

5. Feeling of dizziness, unsteadiness, lightheadedness, or faintness
6. Derealization (feelings of unreality) or depersonalization (self-detachment)
7. Fear of losing control or going crazy; fear of dying; numbness or tingling sensations
8. Chills or hot flashes (American Psychiatric Association, 1994).

Panic Control Treatment (PCT; Barlow & Craske, 1994; Craske & Barlow, 1992) presently constitutes the empirically validated treatment of choice for PD, involving the key components of interoceptive exposure as well as cognitive restructuring (Barlow et al., 1998). Interoceptive exposure confronts the patient with specific physical sensations or symptoms directly associated with his or her panic attacks. For instance, the therapist may have the patient hyperventilate to create shortness of breath or perhaps have the person jog in place to induce sweating and heart rate acceleration. Cognitive restructuring is directed at misconceptions about anxiety and panic (catastrophic cognitions) and distorted cognitions focusing on overestimations of the threat and the danger associated with panic attacks (Barlow et al., 1998).

The application of CBASP as an adjunct to PCT may be especially helpful because it requires the patient to focus specifically on cognitions and behaviors that may be exacerbating symptoms of panic by emphasizing the connection between physical symptoms, thoughts, behaviors, and panic attacks. PCT consists of three main components. The first is a unit of education about the causes and consequences of panic attacks, which is designed to help the patient view panic attacks as less threatening. The second component is exposure to bodily symptoms similar to those present during a panic attack (interoceptive exposure). The third component consists of restructuring cognitions that tend to escalate panic attacks.

No modifications to the CSQ are necessary when incorporating CBASP into PCT, but CBASP should focus on situations specific to having a panic attack or experiencing paniclike symptoms. Emphasis should be placed on those cognitions or interpretations that are specific to the panic symptoms, the events or behaviors before the panic attack occurred, and the patient's behaviors while experiencing panic. Finally, the DO should focus on some aspect of controlling panic, such as evading a panic attack, controlling some of the panic symptoms, reducing the intensity of panic symptoms, and so on.

It is often helpful for the therapist and patient to complete the first CSQs in session so that the patient understands the rationale and purpose of its

7. GENERALIZED ANXIETY DISORDER AND PANIC DISORDER

use in therapy. After that, however, it is important for the patient to complete most of the CSQs as homework. This leaves more time for in-session discussion as well as exposure interventions.

The following case example was derived from our experience with a patient with panic disorder and should help to illustrate how CBASP can be incorporated into PCT.

CASE EXAMPLE 1: PANIC DISORDER

Kara is a 22-year-old undergraduate college student who presented with a concern about a history of panic attacks. Her first panic attack occurred when she was 16 years old, and she experienced two more when she was 19 years old. She stated that these attacks were more than likely precipitated by her use of drugs and alcohol. Kara began experiencing more frequent panic attacks approximately 8 months before seeking treatment and again suspected that some of them might have been due to drug and alcohol use. Although Kara discontinued using drugs and reduced her consumption of alcohol, she continued to experience frequent panic attacks.

When Kara presented for treatment, she was experiencing two or more panic attacks a week. Each generally lasted from several minutes to half an hour. During these episodes, her heart raced, she had difficulty breathing, she had the feeling that her throat was closing up, her stomach felt twisted in knots, and she worried that she was going crazy or was going to die. Kara often experienced panic attacks while at work or when watching an intense movie. Although she reportedly worried about having a panic attack when driving, she did not avoid driving. She also did not avoid work or other social situations in anticipatory fear of a panic attack. Kara did, however, fear having panic attacks when alone at home, and, consequently, she often spent the night at friends' houses.

Based on the information obtained during the intake interview, Kara was diagnosed with PD without Agoraphobia. Accordingly, the treatment plan was to use PCT, Craske and Barlow's (1992) manualized treatment for PD, described previously. In addition, Kara was taught breathing exercises designed to help her manage her level of anxiety during a panic attack. At the outset, CBASP was used in conjunction with PCT to help Kara recognize which physical sensations signaled to her that she was going to have a panic attack, her responses to those sensations, and any thoughts or cognitions escalating or exacerbating her panic attacks. Later in therapy, the CBASP method was used prospectively to help Kara determine which thoughts and behaviors might help her avoid having a panic attack.

The following is a short excerpt of Kara and her therapist working through a CSQ homework assignment in one of these later therapy sessions. Kara had gone to the movies with some friends and began experiencing the symptoms of a panic attack.

Therapist: Did you experience any panic symptoms or panic attacks since our last session?

Kara: Yes—I went to see a horror movie the other night with some of my friends. Halfway through the movie, I began experiencing some panic symptoms.

Therapist: What symptoms specifically?

Kara: My heart started racing, and it was really difficult to breathe. I also started to get a headache.

Therapist: Did you experience a full-blown panic attack at that moment?

Kara: Came close, but I did some of the stuff we talked about before to try and avoid having a full panic attack.

Therapist: The interpretations and behaviors we talked about?

Kara: Yeah.

Therapist: Let's focus first on the thoughts, then. When you started experiencing these panic symptoms in the movie theater, what thoughts helped you avoid having an attack?

Kara: I just kept telling myself, "I am not going to die" and "I can control this."

Therapist: That's great! Do you think that having these thoughts helped you avoid having a panic attack?

Kara: Yeah—they definitely helped me calm down and helped me remember that I was going to be okay and there are other things I can do to keep from having a panic attack.

Therapist: What about your behaviors?

Kara: Well, after I calmed down a little and remembered that I can control this, I started doing the breathing exercises we have been practicing in here. That helped a lot. My heart slowed down and it was easier to breathe.

Clearly, Kara was able to use the skills she had learned from previous sessions to avert a panic attack. Although exposure is the most important component to PCT, recognizing which cognitions and behaviors may lead up to and escalate a panic attack, as well as gener-

7. GENERALIZED ANXIETY DISORDER AND PANIC DISORDER

ating cognitions and behaviors that enable the patient to avoid future panic attacks, is also an important component. In Kara's case, CBASP also helped reveal which behaviors and events led to her panic symptoms. This included consuming large quantities of caffeine earlier in the day, viewing a frightening movie or television show, and extreme stress. When Kara first began experiencing symptoms of a panic attack, such as increased heart rate, shortness of breath and difficulty breathing, she was not able to do anything to control these physical sensations. In addition, when experiencing these symptoms, her thoughts or interpretations were often, "I am going crazy," "I am going to die," and "There is nothing I can do to control this." By obtaining a better understanding of the events, behaviors, and interpretations leading to panic attacks in the context of CBASP assignments, Kara and her therapist were able to devise plans that might enable her to avoid panic attacks. The CSQ was an integral component of this exercise, and the therapist and Kara worked together to generate interpretations and behaviors that would help her evade future panic attacks.

After 20 sessions, Kara's panic symptoms remitted entirely, and her feelings of general anxiety significantly diminished as well. Kara was also able to generalize the skills learned in therapy to address her lack of assertiveness in work and social situations by applying the CBASP methods. These techniques proved effective and Kara reported a significant improvement in her sense of assertiveness.

OBSTACLES TO TREATMENT

One potential obstacle to using the CSQ with PCT is that the patient might not be able to identify specific thoughts that are occurring during a panic attack or just before the attack. In such instances, it is helpful for the therapist to ask the patient to focus on his or her thoughts during interoceptive exposure in session, when panic symptoms, and possibly a panic attack, are being induced in session. This helps the therapist and the patient determine the patient's interpretations before and during a panic attack, on which therapy can later focus to effectively control panic symptoms and avoid future panic attacks.

A second obstacle is that the patient may not understand how the relation of his or her thoughts and behaviors exacerbates symptoms of panic and ultimately leads to a panic attack. If the patient is unable to make this connection, the therapist has to work closely with the patient to help him or her understand how the certain cognitions are connected with behaviors in increasing panic. Fortunately, the CBASP method can be quite useful in this regard as well.

Additionally, after the therapist and patient have determined the cognitions and behaviors involved in escalating panic and alternative thoughts and behaviors to avoid panic, the patient may experience difficulty executing that plan when experiencing panic symptoms. In such cases, it is helpful to try CBASP in session. Again, during interoceptive exposure, remind the patient of the plan (the interpretations and behaviors he or she is to implement to try to avoid a panic attack) and have the patient execute this in session. After receiving support from the therapist—and seeing that the patient has some control—the patient may find it easier to implement the alternate interpretations and behaviors outside of session. It may also be helpful for the therapist to make the patient a note card on which some of the thoughts and behaviors discussed in session are written for the patient's reference when applying CBASP to panic symptoms experienced outside of the therapy room.

Although Kara did not present with symptoms of Agoraphobia, the CSQ can be used in much the same way for the treatment of Agoraphobia. Because the empirically validated treatment for Agoraphobia includes exposure to feared and avoided situations, as well as cognitive restructuring, the therapist can incorporate the CSQ into this treatment as well. Specifically, the patient could complete CSQs that correspond with avoidance behaviors and exposure assignments much in the way CBASP was incorporated into treatment for Social Anxiety Disorder (see Chapter 6, this volume).

In sum, use of CBASP in conjunction with PCT is especially useful for focusing the patient on specific cognitions and behaviors that exacerbate symptoms of panic. It also helps to emphasize the connections between physical symptoms, thoughts, behaviors, and panic attacks.

CBASP APPLICATION TO GENERALIZED ANXIETY DISORDER

According to the *DSM–IV,* the three main diagnostic features of GAD are excessive worry and anxiety about a number of events or activities, occurring more days than not for at least 6 months; extreme difficulty controlling the worry; and persistent overarousal that accompanies the worry. Overarousal can be exhibited several ways, including restlessness or a keyed-up feeling, a feeling of being on edge, fatigue, difficulty concentrating, blank mind, irritability, muscle tension, or sleep disturbance (American Psychiatric Association, 1994). The two principle target components in the treatment of GAD are excessive, uncontrollable worry and persistent overarousal (Brown, O'Leary, & Barlow, 1993). Indeed, although there are fewer treatment outcome studies for GAD, it has been shown that Cognitive Behavioral Therapy (CBT) is superior to behavioral therapy (Butler et al., 1991) and nondirective therapy (Borkovec & Costello, 1993).

Accordingly, the most successful treatments presently available for the treatment of GAD combine exposure, relaxation training, and cognitive therapy, with the goal of bringing the worry process under control (Barlow et al., 1998). This involves exploring irrational anxiety-provoking thoughts and modifying these interpretations by challenging the irrationality of the thoughts. This approach also involves exposure to worry coupled with relaxation (Ballenger, 1999).

As one example, Leahy and Holland's (2000) treatment for GAD prescribes a combination of relaxation training, avoidance confrontation through exposure techniques, worry monitoring, cognitive evaluation of the nature of worrying, interpersonal interventions, stress reduction, and problem-solving training. This approach also calls for distinguishing between productive worry, which results in an immediate plan of action, and unproductive worry, which either does not prompt action or pertains to something outside of one's control. Regardless of type, all worry is postponed until a specified worry time, during which patients are required to ruminate (worry exposure).

As an adjunct to this approach, CBASP enables the therapist and patient to focus specifically on excessive, negative, distorted worries and restructure those worry cognitions. In addition, the therapist and patient are able to focus on any avoidance behaviors or other behaviors that may work to increase worry and anxiety. However, the real benefit of incorporating CBASP into CBT for GAD may be that the CSQ focuses the patient (and therapist) on a specific goal—the DO. It is this focus that illustrates how worries and distorted cognitions, as well as behaviors, may be hurting the patient in his or her effort to achieve a DO (e.g., reduction of worry). The CSQ is also useful in GAD treatment because patients with GAD often cannot focus on a specific worry for a long period of time. They tend to jump from one worry to the other, which maintains their elevated anxiety levels. The purpose of the CSQ is to focus the patient on the thoughts and behaviors that are most helpful in achieving the DO; thus, the CSQ keeps the patient and therapist focused on a specific worry and does not permit the patient to stray to other worries. CBASP teaches patients to maintain a problem-solving, goal-oriented focus rather than unsystematically shifting their attention from one worry to another, which is a typical avoidance mechanism.

As with PCT, no modifications to the CSQ are necessary when incorporating CBASP and the CSQ into CBT for GAD. It can be easily incorporated into Leahy and Holland's (2000) treatment for GAD as an exposure technique, both in session and for in vivo exposure, and for challenging negative thoughts associated with chronic worry. However, when using the CSQ, patients should focus specifically on worry cognitions and behaviors (such as avoidant behaviors) that exacerbate worry and anxiety. The patient's DO should focus on controlling worry, focusing on one topic (or worry) at a time, and reducing anxiety. Once the patient masters the technique and is frequently achieving the DO, the CSQ provides a good source of evidence for challenging remaining worries.

The following case example illustrates the benefit of CBASP for GAD.

CASE EXAMPLE 2: GENERALIZED ANXIETY DISORDER

Michael is a 23-year-old college student who presented with concerns about excessive and uncontrollable worry. He came to our clinic after having a severe anxiety attack, difficulty controlling worry, and thoughts of suicide. At the beginning of therapy, he indicated a moderate level of depression (Beck Depression Inventory = 15), a high level of anxiety (Beck Anxiety Inventory = 27), and clinical elevations on the Minnesota Multiphasic Personality Inventory–2 scales for depression, psychasthenia (anxiety), and social isolation.

At intake, Michael indicated that his excessive worry was mostly concentrated on academic and social failures. He disclosed that the primary stressors that led to his anxiety attack included an unanticipated increase in his academic workload, feelings of total isolation, and lack of social support. Michael's worry consumed much of his day and typically focused on small, unrelated matters, such as his gait and his perceived lack of table etiquette. Michael's anxiety manifested

7. GENERALIZED ANXIETY DISORDER AND PANIC DISORDER

in his self-proclaimed feelings of being keyed up and on edge, which was very apparent in his early sessions.

Michael was diagnosed with GAD and Obsessive-Compulsive Personality Disorder (e.g., preoccupation with lists and details, perfectionism, overly conscientious about morality, and reluctance to delegate work). The treatment plan included CBT for GAD as outlined in Leahy and Holland (2000) with the integration of CBASP and the CSQ. The goal of this treatment plan was to identify and challenge any cognitive distortions and the attendant behaviors maintaining Michael's worry and anxiety to help him develop a more realistic, goal-oriented approach to his behavior. When Michael came to our clinic he was engaging in extensive exercise that included aerobics and weight lifting. He rarely consumed caffeine or alcoholic beverages. The therapist, therefore, decided to direct primary attention to the cognitive and behavioral components of the treatment plan and to implement additional relaxation techniques as necessary.

The CSQ was used to decrease Michael's avoidant social behaviors. Michael spent an inordinate amount of time worrying about how others perceived him (e.g., "if I'm out alone people will think that I'm pathetic"). His incessant worry about others' perceptions of him often interfered with his engagement in pleasurable activities and his initiation and maintenance of meaningful and intimate relationships. The CSQ aided Michael in working through his negative thoughts in session, and he was given exposure homework assignments that further addressed specific worries. For example, although Michael enjoyed going to the movie theater, he would not go alone and feared rejection if he asked someone to accompany him. After working through a CSQ focusing on this worry, Michael was given an exposure homework assignment that required that he ask someone out to a movie, and go to the movie, even if the person he asked refused to accompany him.

The CSQ is also useful in noninterpersonal situations (e.g., worry about academic failures). Michael had recurrent dreams about failing a high school class, and his worst possible outcome was that he would be unsuccessful in his career. Michael's compensatory strategy for reducing his fear of failure (i.e., taking on too many tasks) had the opposite effect. Rather than reducing anxiety and worry about failure, Michael's compensatory strategy created more stress and time pressure, in which anxiety and worry were much more likely to occur.

Michael worried daily about task completion, which often led to his use of procrastination and distraction as coping mechanisms. The following is a CSQ taken from an early session in which the CSQ was useful in delineating how Michael's thoughts and behaviors were working against him.

Elicitation Phase

Situation:
Michael had spent a stressful and frustrating night working on a project that was due the following morning. He started working on the project around 9 P.M. and completed it at 8 A.M. the following morning.

Interpretations:
God, I am such a slacker. . . . I should have done this earlier. . . . This is all my fault. . . . I could have prevented this. . . . I'm doing this much slower than everyone else. . . . Is this what graduate school will be like?

Behaviors:
Pounded on desk. . . . Paced because I couldn't concentrate. . . . Took a break and watched television for a few hours.

Desired Outcome:
I wanted to work faster and complete the project by 1 A.M.

Actual Outcome:
I was up all night working on the project.

Clearly, Michael's cognitions were not conducive to achieving his goal and diminished his ability to focus on the task at hand. After discussing whether Michael's interpretations were helpful or hurtful with regards to achieving his DO, he produced the following interpretations and behaviors that would have increased the likelihood of his DO.

Remediation

Interpretations:
This is not an impossible task. . . . This is taking longer to complete than I expected, but I am making progress, and if

7. GENERALIZED ANXIETY DISORDER AND PANIC DISORDER   113

I continue to work on it, I will finish it. . . . In order to finish this on time, I need to stay in the moment and concentrate on this task.

Behaviors:
Work in 1-hr time blocks and take shorter breaks. Do not turn on the television.

Therapist: Michael, how would it have helped you to complete the project by 1:00 A.M. if you had thought, "This is taking much longer to complete than I planned, but I am making progress, and if I continue to work on it I will finish it?"

Michael: It may not have helped me finish it by 1 A.M., but I don't think I would have been so frustrated if I had realized the amount of progress I was making and had concentrated on finishing it instead of everything else that was going on in my head. And I probably wouldn't have watched television so long if I hadn't been so upset, and I would have finished sooner than 8 A.M.

Therapist: It sounds like you're saying that your DO may not have been realistic given the circumstances.

Michael: So you're saying that I put more pressure on myself by saying that I had to finish by 1:00 A.M.?

Therapist: Is that what happened?

Michael: Yes, I think so. I know that I didn't plan this out very well. I knew about this assignment well in advance but kept putting it off.

Therapist: Do you do that a lot, put things off until the last minute?

Michael: Yes.

Therapist: Why do you think that is?

Michael: Sometimes I just underestimate the amount of time it takes me to do things, and sometimes I put things off because thinking about them makes me more anxious.

Therapist: It's good that you realize that part of your procrastination is related to your anxiety. Based on the CSQ that we've just worked through, how do you think your procrastination affects your worry and anxiety?

Michael: I don't know. It seems that when I put things off until the last minute, even though I feel better when I'm not thinking about it, in the long run it makes me more anxious and affects the thoughts I have about myself.

Therapist: What do you mean?

Michael: Well, if I hadn't put this assignment off, I wouldn't be thinking that I'm a slacker or that I am a failure.

Therapist: Good. Do you think working through this situation will help you in similar situations in the future?

Michael: Definitely. First I don't think that I will put things off until the very last minute, but if I do, I know that it's important to direct all my attention to the task at hand, and thinking about what should or could have happened is not productive in the moment.

This transcript provides a clear demonstration of the use of the CSQ technique for redirecting GAD patients' attention away from negative thoughts and toward goal-directed thoughts and behaviors. It is clear that although Michael's initial thoughts did not help him get his DO, through remediation he was able to generate alternative thoughts. He was further able to recognize that given the circumstances, his initial DO was neither realistic nor attainable.

As this example illustrates, the CSQ provides the therapist with a useful exposure tool, while also allowing for simultaneous challenge of negative thoughts and avoidant behavior. Following his 10th session of CBASP, Michael's anxiety and tension had significantly decreased (Beck Anxiety Inventory = 6) and he no longer avoided engaging in enjoyable activities because of others' perceptions. Indeed, Michael expressed his surprise at not having anything to worry about during worry time.

OBSTACLES TO TREATMENT

Incorporation of the CSQ into the CBT treatment for GAD was made easier by two of the patient's characteristics, intelligence and motivation. Whereas it typically takes patients several sessions to get a firm grasp of the connection between their thoughts, behaviors, and outcomes, Michael almost immediately made the connection. Within the first few sessions, he started to apply the concept on his own and never needed to be prompted or reminded to provide a CSQ for each session. Although not all patients make such speedy progress, steady therapeutic gains can be expected with motivated patients, regardless of intelligence level.

An obstacle to applying CBASP to the treatment of GAD is the distress and anxious arousal that some patients feel. This may leave them unable or unwilling to focus on the content of the worry. Thus, instead of focusing on worry specific to one content area, they may focus on worries in multiple content areas to reduce the anxiety related to a specific worry. This can be problematic because CBASP is goal oriented and requires the patient and therapist to focus on one content area at a time (this is also a requirement of the worry exposure component of CBT for GAD; see Brown, O'Leary, & Barlow, 1993). In addition, anxious arousal may keep the patient from engaging in exposure exercises and discussion of the CSQs. It is therefore helpful to teach relaxation techniques and use these techniques in session (or outside of session) when the patient experiences high levels of anxious arousal that interfere with the therapeutic process and in completing the CSQ exercise.

In this chapter, we outlined the incorporation of McCullough's (2000) CBASP, particularly the use of the CSQ, into empirically validated CBT for PD (with or without agoraphobia) and GAD. The CSQ provides a goal-oriented, problem-solving, focused approach critical to making therapeutic gains with these disorders. For PD, this goal involves the reduction in, or cessation of, panic symptoms and panic attacks, whereas for GAD the DO is a reduction in worrisome thinking and overall anxiety levels. For both PD and GAD, the CSQ can be used both concurrently and prospectively.

Although this chapter discussed in detail how CBASP can be applied to CBT for PD and GAD and offered case examples from our clinic to illustrate its successful implementation, it should be kept in mind that this method has not yet been empirically validated. CBASP, however, is an empirically validated treatment with depression, and thus its incorporation into empirically validated treatments for PD and GAD should only enhance the efficacy of established interventions for these disorders.

PART III

Parents, Children, and Couples

Chapter **8**

Parents of Children Diagnosed With Behavior Disorders*

> Parents of children with behavior disorders often focus on the need to change the child's behavior without recognizing the role that their own thoughts and behaviors play in the perpetuation of family conflicts. This chapter summarizes existing empirically validated treatments for externalizing behavior disorders and argues for the incorporation of the Cognitive Behavioral Analysis System of Psychotherapy into these treatments. The unmodified use of the Cognitive Behavioral Analysis System with parents in a group therapy setting is demonstrated to be an effective means for positively changing parents' thoughts and behaviors, resulting in improvement not only in children's behaviors but also in overall family functioning.

Due to the disruptive nature of externalizing behaviors, conduct disorders are the most frequently cited problem in both clinic-referred and general populations (Quay, 1986). Externalizing behavior includes aggressive, antisocial, and noncompliant acts that are subsumed by the childhood syndromes Attention-Deficit/Hyperactivity Disorder (ADHD), Oppositional Defiant Disorder (ODD) and Conduct Disorder (CD).

ADHD is characterized by multiple symptoms of inattention, impulsivity, or both, that are developmentally incongruent. These symptoms must be present in multiple settings (e.g., school, social, and home) for at least 6 months, resulting in significant impairment. Although this disorder does

---

*The primary authors contributing to this chapter were Rebecca R. Gerhardstein, Rita Ketterman, and Scharles C. Petty.

not assume aggressive or antisocial behavior, ADHD is frequently co-morbid with CD (American Psychiatric Association, 1994). Multimodal treatment of ADHD is suggested, including stimulant medication, Parent Management Training (PMT), and school-based interventions focused on classroom behavior and academic performance (Tripp & Sutherland, 1999).

The *Diagnostic and Statistical Manual of Mental Disorders–Fourth Edition* (*DSM–IV;* American Psychiatric Association, 1994) lists two categories of disruptive behavior disorders: ODD and CD. The essential feature of ODD is a recurrent pattern of negativistic, defiant, disobedient, and hostile behavior toward authority figures characterized by the frequent occurrence of losing one's temper, arguing with adults, active noncompliance, and deliberate annoyance of others. CD is characterized by a persistent pattern of behavior in which the rights of others and age-appropriate social norms are violated. The critical distinction between these two disorders is that ODD behaviors are less severe in nature and typically do not include aggression toward people or animals, destruction of property, theft, or deceit. Patients with earlier onset of CD are characterized by behavior that is more aggressive in nature, whereas adolescent onset reflects more delinquent behavior, such as vandalism and theft (American Psychiatric Association, 1994). Antisocial behavior (ASB) is defined by acts that reflect social rule violations and actions against others. A wide range of ASB is highly correlated with child, parent, and family functioning that could be considered conduct-disordered behavior (e.g., substance use and association with delinquent peers); however, CD is considered beyond ASB in its frequency, intensity, and chronicity, which results in impairment of the child's ability to function (Kazdin, 1997).

The multiple factors and pathways that contribute to the etiology of these disruptive behavior syndromes make it difficult to determine the exact relationships between them (American Psychiatric Association, 1994; Kazdin, 1997). Child-centered factors (e.g., temperament, neurological, cognitive and intellectual deficits), parental factors (e.g., birth complications, family history of psychopathology, punishment and parenting practices, supervision of child, marital discord), and environmental factors (e.g., family size, socioeconomic disadvantage, school setting) interact with each other to influence the development of externalizing behavior on a continuum from ODD to CD (Kazdin 1998). The *DSM–IV* (American Psychiatric Association, 1994) diagnosis of CD subsumes the symptoms of ODD, reflecting the belief that one disorder may be a sufficient, but not a necessary, developmental link to the other. In addition, these risk factors

TREATMENTS FOR EXTERNALIZING BEHAVIORS

There are several empirically based treatments for externalizing behaviors: PMT, Cognitive Problem-Solving Skills Training (PSST), and multisystemic therapy (MST). Each of these treatments has repeatedly demonstrated efficacy in controlled trials with follow-up periods of at least 1 year in children with behavior severe enough to warrant referral to clinical settings (Kazdin, 2000).

In PMT, it is assumed that behavior problems in the child will be reduced if parents change the reinforcement contingencies that maintain deviant behavior. The techniques used in PMT are taught to parents to alter their interactions with their children to reduce coercive interactions (Kazdin, 2000). Treatment typically includes principles of behavior management and specific skills training, such as attending, rewarding, ignoring, giving directions, giving time out, and maintaining token economies when appropriate (Brosnan & Carr, 2000; Tripp & Sutherland, 1999). The PMT paradigm indirectly adopts a systems perspective (Estrada & Pinsof, 1995), which is important because many familial characteristics, such as psychopathology, criminal behavior, substance abuse, harsh punishment practices, poor supervision, poor relationships within family, marital discord, larger family size, low socioeconomic status (SES), and an older sibling with ASB, are each correlated with externalizing behaviors (Kazdin, 1997).

PSST is aimed at correcting the cognitive distortions and deficiencies that have been associated with teacher ratings of disruptive behavior, peer evaluations, and direct assessment of overt behavior in a variety of settings. Examples of such impaired cognitive processes include the generation of alternative solutions to interpersonal problems, the planning and implementation of steps necessary to achieve a goal, the recognition of consequences related to one's own actions, the perception of how others feel, and the interpretion of others' motivations for their actions. Children are taught to examine their thought processes that guide their behavior in interpersonal situations. Self-statements are taught to enable them to direct attention to situational cues that lead to effective solutions. Furthermore, the results of the child's behavior are also examined to identify and reinforce prosocial behavior (Kazdin, 2000).

MST takes a holistic approach to the treatment of externalizing behavior through the examination of family, peer, school, and neighborhood systems in search of the variables that lead to the development, maintenance, or amelioration of problematic behavior. MST examines the bidirectional interaction between the child and his or her environment, with a specific focus on how the child's behavior affects others. This treatment has been used primarily with delinquent adolescents. The treatment goals are broad and may include helping parents to develop the adolescent's prosocial behavior and helping them resolve marital conflicts that undermine parenting and reduce cohesion among family members. The techniques used to accomplish this include PMT, contingency management, PSST, and marital therapy (Kazdin, 2000).

Of the empirically validated treatments for externalizing behaviors, PMT has been evaluated the most frequently through numerous randomized, controlled outcome trials with children ranging in age from 2 to 17 years, across a continuum of severity of conduct-disordered behavior. Brestan and Eyberg's (1998) review named PMT as the only well-established treatment for CD. PMT led to such vast improvement in children's behavior that nonclinical, normative levels were obtained through ratings by both parents and teachers, through direct observation of behavior at home and school, and through examination of institutional records. Often such gains were maintained from 1 to 3 years, and in one study they were maintained from 10 to 14 years posttreatment. In addition, indirect treatment effects were in improved sibling behavior in the home and decreased depression and other psychopathology. The theoretical foundation of PMT is strongly based in family systems and interpersonal dynamics, principles of social learning theory, and behavioral analysis (Kazdin, 2000). For these reasons, PMT was determined to be the treatment of choice for parents of children exhibiting externalizing behavior at our clinic.

However, the limitations of PMT were also considered. As with any treatment, the patient must agree that the intervention offered is valuable, applicable, and effective. Parental commitment to the intervention facilitates consistent attendance, consistent practice of the observation of the child's behavior, consistent implementation, and consistent supervision of reward and punishment schedules to increase the likelihood of positive outcomes. This may not be easily accomplished because parents frequently

8. PARENTS OF CHILDREN WITH BEHAVIOR DISORDERS

see the child's behavior as the problem and point of intervention, rather than the aforementioned risk factors, which include parenting practices. In addition, the amount of social learning theory and reinforcement principles that parents must master to stop the coercive cycle and reduce the escalation of conflict between family members, improve the family environment, and increase the child's prosocial behavior may be daunting (Kazdin, 2000). Lastly, a direct problem-solving skills component is not delineated in PMT, despite the success of PSST with parents of children with externalizing behavior problems.

The incorporation of CBASP (McCullough, 2000) offers a potential solution to these limitations. CBASP provides a concrete, systematic method of observation and analysis of both parental and child behavior that leads to the identification of the antecedents and consequences of behavior, as well as natural reinforcers and punishers. The ability to educate parents in the use of CBASP at home increases their consistency in observation. Analysis of behavior in both problematic and nonproblematic situations effectively teaches the principles and importance of social learning theory, while providing reinforcement with highly salient, personalized examples. Problem-solving skills are also taught and increased through use of CBASP. In addition, its use promotes the implementation and supervision of behavior schedules. Lastly, CBASP is very portable. It is a skill that parents can learn and apply in any situation, at any time, thereby decreasing the negative impact of poor therapy attendance and attrition.

Two manualized PMT treatments by Bloomquist (1996) and Barkley (1997) were combined with CBASP to produce the treatment used in our clinic with parents of children who engaged in externalizing behaviors.

INCORPORATION OF CBASP INTO PMT

Bloomquist (1996) and Barkley (1997) offer training for parents of children with externalizing behavior disorders, such as ADHD, ODD, and CD. Barkley focuses primarily on teaching parents reinforcement strategies to help improve their child's aversive behavior (e.g., forgetting their homework at school, yelling out answers in class), whereas Bloomquist focuses primarily on teaching parents methods for improving their children's social skills (e.g., demonstrating techniques for how to initiate a conversation with an unknown child). In addition, Bloomquist offers a section that helps parents manage their own stress and teaches them how to monitor their negative thoughts. The notion of teaching parents how to monitor and perhaps even change their thoughts is consistent with the notion that parents need to learn how to manage themselves before they can help their children to do so.

In addition to these beneficial interventions, CBASP offers a relatively simple format for integrating the cognitive and behavioral teachings of Barkley (1997) and Bloomquist (1996). In the first step (situation), parents describe a specific situation in which their child is noncompliant. In the second step (thoughts), parents describe the thoughts that they are having during the situation. In the third step (behaviors), parents describe what they did in the situation (e.g., how they acted, how they appeared to others, what they said). In the fourth step (Actual Outcome, or AO), parents describe the outcome of the situation. In the fifth and final step (Desired Outcome, or DO), parents describe how they would have liked the situation to turn out for them. Typically, the AOs and DOs do not match. After parents realize that they did not get what they wanted, the real intervention occurs in the remediation of Steps 2 (thoughts) and 3 (behaviors). During this process, the focus is on the identification of helpful or hurtful thoughts and behaviors relative to their DO. Should a thought or behavior be labeled as hurtful, an alternative, helpful thought or behavior is identified.

In most cases, the helpful thoughts or behaviors come directly from Bloomquist's and Barkley's manuals. Bloomquist (1996) suggested that when a parent thinks "My child is behaving like a brat" an alternative thought would be "My child behaves positively, too." CBASP offers a framework to this process by focusing on how a thought was hurtful and how changing a hurtful thought to a helpful one aids in the achievement of the parents' DO. Focusing on what parents ideally want from interactions with their children motivates them to think about how their thoughts are impacting their behavior and, in turn, the outcome of these interactions. This motivates parents to change their thoughts and behaviors to have a positive impact on the interactions with their children.

Barkley (1997) offers many examples of how parents can help shape their child's behavior, such as rewarding good behavior and ignoring bad behavior. In many cases this is extremely difficult to do. For example, when parents determine a punishment for their child and the child throws a tantrum, the parents may give in and relinquish the punishment. Inadvertently, the parents have just negatively reinforced their child for throwing a temper tantrum (Barkley, 1997). Negative reinforcement is often difficult for parents to conceptualize; however, it can be directly illustrated using

CBASP. In the analysis of a specific situation, the therapist asks whether the parents' behavior of removing the punishment helped them achieve the DO. The recognition that specific parental behaviors are not working, though difficult to admit, is perhaps an easier concept to grasp than abstract principles of reinforcement. After the parents recognize that removing the punishment prevented them from achieving their DO, they may be able to see that consistent punishment and ignoring the child's tantrum would be more helpful in attaining the DO.

Reinforcement, punishment, and social learning principles are the basis of the incorporation of CBASP into PMT, and these principles are illustrated in specific situations that are more salient to parents. Specifically, helpful thoughts and behaviors that parents can ultimately perform to achieve goals are identified. CBASP is consistent with the concepts advocated by Bloomquist (1996) and Barkley (1997), and it provides a vehicle by which in-depth illustration of social learning principles can occur in a way that is meaningful and nonthreatening to parents. Because the understanding of social learning principles is related to better treatment outcomes (Kazdin, 1997), the incorporation of CBASP into PMT may increase treatment effectiveness.

The incorporation of CBASP into PMT also reduces parents' tendency to use session time to complain, which is nonproductive. The specificity in Step 1 and the changing of parental thoughts and behaviors in Steps 2 and 3 motivate change by forcing parents to focus on what they want and on methods that will help them to achieve those outcomes. Also, the systematic framework that CBASP affords is likely to increase consistency in parental behavior, which is frequently cited as key to improved parenting and increased desired behavior in children (Bloomquist, 1996).

An added benefit of CBASP is that it is the crux of an empirically validated technique used in chronic depression (Keller et al., 2000). Many parents who have struggled to deal with difficult children report depressive symptoms (Bloomquist, 1996). CBASP was devised to help patients counter negative thoughts that exacerbate or maintain depression. The same technique can be used to help parents become aware of negative evaluations that are made about their children, their parenting skills, their circumstances, and their spouse or themselves. It can also be used not only to illustrate the relationships in the immediate situation but also to emphasize the long-term emotional consequences of harboring such beliefs.

Many benefits of using CBASP with parents of children with ADHD, ODD, or CD have been observed in session. As with most psychosocial treatments, the outcome of PMT is affected by the duration of treatment (Kazdin, 1997). Often, parental resistance to PMT results in reduced in-session participation, treatment dissatisfaction, and parental noncompliance (Estrada & Pinsof, 1995). Treatment noncompliance is likely increased by the presence of parental characteristics that have been associated with the development and maintenance of externalizing behavior in children, such as harsh, lax, erratic, and inconsistent disciplinary practices; alcoholism; criminal behavior; marital discord; interpersonal conflict and inequality; and aggression. In addition, relationships between the parent and child may be less accepting, less warm, less affectionate, and less emotionally supportive, which results in reduced attachment and interaction (Kazdin, 1997). The analysis of thoughts and behaviors may illuminate family dynamics that may affect treatment effectiveness, and consideration should be given to handling these issues in individual or couples sessions. In addition, CBASP enables the therapist to confront ineffectual parental and interpersonal behavior in an indirect manner, which decreases resistance.

Importantly, the CBASP technique of problem solving can be taught to children as well as parents (see Chapter 9, this volume). The technique becomes, in effect, a common operating system that allows parents and children to discuss problematic interpersonal interactions in a nonjudgmental, nonconfrontational manner. Anecdotal evidence shows that the application of CBASP in this manner reduces escalation of emotion and reinforces lessons taught in session. Lastly, prospective use of CBASP can be helpful in anticipation of situations where misbehavior is likely to occur. Parents and children can be taught to start with their DO and determine the thoughts and behaviors that increase the likelihood of obtaining satisfactory results.

BRIEF DESCRIPTION OF GROUP THERAPY

Conducting PMT in group settings in not uncommon. There are several benefits to the group therapy approach. First, it helps with treatment compliance to see other parents regularly bringing in homework. It creates social pressure for any negligent parents to bring in their homework as well. In addition, many parents find it useful to hear others discussing their implementation of the principles of both CBASP and PMT. Not only can they relate to the problematic situations that other parents bring up, but

8. PARENTS OF CHILDREN WITH BEHAVIOR DISORDERS

also they can learn from other parents' mistakes and successes. Moreover, when a parent is struggling with the steps of CBASP, it is invaluable if there are other parents available to offer suggestions about alternative thoughts and behaviors that may have been helpful in the situation.

For each case the adult group followed a 12-week itinerary stressing an integration of Bloomquist (1996), Barkley (1997), and McCullough's (2000) techniques. Although the following cases and treatment plan are examples of the combination of CBASP and PMT in a group setting, it is possible that they can be applied to individual cases as well. The Coping Skills Questionnaire (CSQ) is the primary tool by which CBASP is implemented in this approach. It consists of a single sheet of paper (assigned for homework every week), which lists the five steps of CBASP (i.e., situation, thoughts, behaviors, AO, and DO). An outline of the group format is shown in Table 8.1.

To best illustrate the integration of CBASP and PMT, two case examples are presented. Both families attended simultaneous parent and child groups offered at our clinic: one group was for parents only and one for children only. (For a complete description of the child group, see

TABLE 8.1
Outline of Group Format

Week	Description of Activities
Week 1	Introduction and Chapter 3 from Bloomquist (1996) Discussion of stress management, the coercive cycle, and consistency Homework: Work on stress management techniques
Week 2	Review consistency and Chapter 4 from Bloomquist (1996) Introduction of McCullough's Coping Skills Questionnaire (CSQ) Steps 1 through 5 Discussion of changing hurtful thoughts into helpful thoughts, including an integration of Bloomquist's Chapter 4 and McCullough's Step 2 of the CSQ (thoughts) The impact of Step 2 of the CSQ (thoughts) on Steps 4 and 5 (outcomes) is considered. Homework: Complete a CSQ
Week 3	Review consistency and review the CSQ Each parent's CSQ homework is considered within the group. Should any parent have difficulty changing hurtful thoughts to helpful thoughts, the group is consulted. Homework: Complete a CSQ

(Continued)

TABLE 8.1 *(Continued)*

Week	Description of Activities
Week 4	Review consistency, the CSQ, and Steps 2 and 3 from Barkley (1997) Each parent's CSQ is considered within the group. Discussion of Step 3 of the CSQ (changing hurtful behaviors into helpful behaviors) follows with an emphasis on the techniques from Steps 2 and 3 from Barkley (paying attention and rewarding good behavior). The impact of Step 3 of the CSQ (behaviors) on Steps 4 and 5 (outcomes) is considered. Homework: Complete a CSQ
Week 5	Review consistency and the CSQ Each parent's CSQ homework is considered within the group. Should any parent have difficulty changing hurtful behaviors into helpful behaviors, the group is consulted. Homework: Complete a CSQ
Week 6	Review consistency, the CSQ, and Step 5 from Barkley (1997) Each parent's CSQ is considered within the group. Discussion of Step 3 of the CSQ (changing hurtful behaviors into helpful behaviors) follows with an emphasis on the techniques from Step 5 of Barkley (ignoring bad behavior). The impact of Step 3 of the CSQ (behaviors) on Steps 4 and 5 (outcomes) is considered. Homework: Complete a CSQ
Week 7	Review consistency and the CSQ Each parent's CSQ homework is considered within the group. Should any parent have difficulty changing hurtful thoughts and behaviors into helpful thoughts and behaviors, the group is consulted. Homework: Complete a CSQ
Week 8	Review the CSQ and Step 4 from Barkley (1997) Each parent's CSQ is considered within the group. Discussion of Steps 2 and 3 of the CSQ (changing hurtful thoughts and behaviors into helpful thoughts and behaviors) follows. The impact of Steps 2 and 3 of the CSQ on Steps 4 and 5 (outcomes) is considered. Barkley's Step 4 (token economy) is reviewed as a method for consistently rewarding good behavior and ignoring bad behavior within the home. Homework: Complete a CSQ, consider token economy

(Continued)

8. PARENTS OF CHILDREN WITH BEHAVIOR DISORDERS 129

TABLE 8.1 *(Continued)*

Week	Description of Activities
Week 9	Review CSQ and token economy Each parent's CSQ is considered within the group. Discussion of Steps 2 and 3 of the CSQ (changing hurtful thoughts and behaviors into helpful thoughts and behaviors) follows. The impact of Steps 2 and 3 of the CSQ on Steps 4 and 5 (outcomes) is considered. Problem solving the implementation of Barkley's token economy within the household is reviewed. Homework: Complete a CSQ
Week 10	Review the CSQ and Step 8 from Barkley (1997) Each parent's CSQ is considered within the group. Discussion of Steps 2 and 3 of the CSQ (changing hurtful thoughts and behaviors into helpful thoughts and behaviors) follows. The impact of Steps 2 and 3 of the CSQ on Steps 4 and 5 (outcomes) is considered. Barkley's Step 8 (behavioral report card) is reviewed as a method for consistently rewarding good behavior and ignoring bad behavior within the classroom environment. Homework: Complete a CSQ and consider the behavioral report card
Week 11	Review the CSQ and the behavioral report card Each parent's CSQ is considered within the group. Discussion of Steps 2 and 3 of the CSQ (changing hurtful thoughts and behaviors into helpful thoughts and behaviors) follows. The impact of Steps 2 and 3 of the CSQ on Steps 4 and 5 (outcomes) is considered. Problem solving the implementation of Barkley's behavioral report card within the classroom environment is reviewed. Homework: Complete a CSQ
Week 12	Review the CSQ and Chapter 6 from Bloomquist (1996) Each parent's CSQ is considered within the group. Discussion of Steps 2 and 3 of the CSQ (changing hurtful thoughts and behaviors into helpful thoughts and behaviors) follows. The impact of Steps 2 and 3 of the CSQ on Steps 4 and 5 (outcomes) is considered. Bloomquist's strategies for positive familial interactions are reviewed. Parents are encouraged to continue using the CSQ on their own.

Chapter 9, this volume.) Prior to both families' attendance at the first group session, they completed interviews to determine the presenting problem and to determine whether they were considered appropriate additions to the groups.

⟶ CASE EXAMPLE 1 ⟵

Susan is a 39-year-old mother of three. Her daughter Gretchen is 10 years old and the middle child in her family. Gretchen's father lives with them at home but was not a part of treatment. Susan first brought Gretchen to the clinic because she wanted help teaching Gretchen peer relation skills. Susan also wanted to reduce Gretchen's frequent emotional outbursts, which were beginning to interfere not only with Gretchen's relationships with her friends but also with her relationships at home. Gretchen received a diagnosis of ODD and was referred to the child group. Susan was not diagnosed, but it was clear from her interview that she was experiencing depressed mood and chronic stress related to the problems that she was having with Gretchen. Susan was referred to the corresponding adult group. The following is a transcript of an unsuccessful CSQ with Susan.

Unsuccessful CSQ

> *Step 1:* Situation
>> I asked Gretchen if she thought it was time for bed, and we ended up getting into an argument about her bedtime. She was trying everything she could to get me to agree to let her stay up. I was getting angry, and she was throwing a temper tantrum.

> *Step 2:* Thoughts
>> She knows exactly what to say to me to get me angry.
>> I must be a very bad mother because I don't know how to get her to stop.
>> Maybe I should just let her have it her way and enforce my rules next time.

> *Step 3:* Behaviors
>> I yelled some more but got so tired of our argument that I gave in and let her stay up another 30 min.

8. PARENTS OF CHILDREN WITH BEHAVIOR DISORDERS

Step 4: AO
  Gretchen stopped yelling, but she didn't go to bed on time.
  I didn't enforce my rules.

Step 5: DO
  I wanted Gretchen to stop yelling at me. I wanted her to go to
  bed on time like I had told her. I really wish I hadn't yelled at
  Gretchen and that I could enforce my rules without yelling.

When discussing Susan's CSQ, the group decided to focus on Susan's DO of enforcing rules without yelling. It was determined that none of Susan's thoughts were helping her to calmly enforce her rules. Examples of some alternative thoughts were suggested, such as "If I give in to her this time, the next time I want Gretchen to do something she will be less likely to do it" and "Remain calm. Yelling at Gretchen is not going to make her any more likely to go to bed." The group determined that both of these thoughts would likely help Susan to enforce her rules without yelling. In addition, the group decided that Susan's behavior of letting Gretchen stay up later was not helping Susan enforce her rules. Instead, it was suggested that Susan escort Gretchen to her bed and turn off the lights; remove distractions, such as television and video games; speak in a calm nononsense voice telling (not asking) Gretchen that it is time for bed. Finally, Susan and the group were asked whether Susan would have been more likely to get what she wanted if she had used the alternative thoughts and behaviors. The group agreed that she probably would have gotten what she wanted using helpful thoughts and actions.

The following are Susan's responses on a successful CSQ.

Successful CSQ

Step 1: Situation
  Gretchen and I were driving in the car, and she was really irritating me. She was being loud and kicking the back of my seat really hard. I told her to stop, and she did not stop. I was getting more and more angry at her.

Step 2: Thoughts
  I thought she was being a complete brat.

Wait, remember what we have talked about in group? You can control your own thoughts and behaviors. You know what to do.
Relax. Ignore her. She will stop.

Step 3: Behaviors
I stopped the car and turned the radio off and didn't say another word to her.

Step 4: AO
This was the first time that I actually got what I wanted. I controlled my reaction to my daughter. The really cool thing was that by controlling my reaction to Gretchen, I impacted her behavior, too (she stopped).

Step 5: DO
I really wanted Gretchen to stop kicking my seat, but I know that I couldn't completely control that. What I wanted for myself was to control my reaction to her (not yell, not swerve on the road).

Throughout the course of treatment, Susan made a great deal of progress with her ability to evaluate her thoughts and behaviors. This example represents the first time that she actually employed the CSQ while she was in a situation. After weeks of considering the helpfulness of her thoughts and actions post hoc, she finally took the much-needed step and applied the CSQ techniques during the situation. She excitedly brought this CSQ back to the group and was met with many accolades. Because of this reinforcement, she continued to use the CSQ technique for the remainder of the group sessions.

CASE EXAMPLE 2

Cheryl is a 45-year-old mother of three. Nathan is 12 years old and the youngest child in his family. Nathan's stepfather lives with them at home, but was not a part of the group treatment. Cheryl first brought her son Nathan to the clinic because of problems with anger control, class disruption, social problems, and academic difficulties. She wanted an evaluation and possibly therapy for her son. Nathan received a diagnosis of ADHD and ODD and was referred to the child

8. PARENTS OF CHILDREN WITH BEHAVIOR DISORDERS   133

group. Cheryl was not diagnosed, but it was clear from her interview that she was experiencing depressed mood and chronic stress related to the problems that she was having with Nathan. Cheryl was referred to the corresponding adult group. In addition, both mother and son were receiving individual therapy. Cheryl's responses on an unsuccessful CSQ follow.

Unsuccessful CSQ

Step 1: Situation

Nathan was not listening to me. I asked him repeatedly to clean up his room, and he was watching TV instead. I found myself getting more and more angry at him.

Step 2: Thoughts

He was driving me absolutely crazy.

If he doesn't make some movement toward his room really soon, I am going to grab him and shake him until he listens to me.

Maybe if I stand right next to him and yell in his ear, he will do what I want him to do.

Step 3: Behaviors

I yelled at him, saying, "If you don't clean up your room right now, you are going to get a whooping."

I ran and got my paddle and waved it in front of his face.

Step 4: AO

Nathan cleaned his room but only after I yelled and threatened him. I got really angry. I'll bet my blood pressure went up 30 points!

Step 5: DO

I wanted Nathan to listen to me on the first try. I wanted him to obey me and not make me angry. I wanted to not let him have so much control over my emotions. I wanted Nathan to clean his room.

When reviewing the CSQ, the group realized that Cheryl has very little control over any of her DOs. They asked her to determine whether there were any realistic DOs with which Cheryl could be satisfied. She settled on the outcome of not losing her self-control (i.e., not yelling, not waving the paddle in front of Nathan's face). It was determined that none of Cheryl's thoughts were helping her maintain her composure. Some alternative thoughts were generated, such as "I need to relax before I speak with Nathan," "Maybe I should practice some of my stress management techniques," and "My touching Nathan is not going to help me remain calm; he will likely fight back and I will really lose control then." These thoughts focused on the consequences of Cheryl's actions, which could help her maintain her composure when dealing with Nathan. In addition, the group decided that yelling and waving the paddle in front of Nathan's face was not helping her maintain self-control. Instead, the group suggested that Cheryl remove herself from the situation and employ a stress management technique. Cheryl and the rest of the group agreed that she probably would have gotten what she wanted if she had used more helpful thoughts and behaviors.

Successful CSQ

> *Step 1:* Situation
>> Nathan misplaced a toy. I let him look around for it on his own, but he gave up saying, "Never mind. I can't find it." I volunteered to help him look for his toy, but he yelled at me saying, "You don't trust me. You must think I'm stupid."

> *Step 2:* Thoughts
>> This toy has to be somewhere; he just got it today.
>> Nathan thinks that this is all my fault, and he's mad at me.
>> Whoa! I'm doing that again! Cut it out. It's not your fault.
>> This is not worth getting worked up over.

> *Step 3:* Behaviors
>> I really thought about yelling back at him that I do love him and trust him, but I held my tongue. Instead, I simply said that I do trust him; I stopped looking for the toy and went back to my work.

> *Step 4:* AO
>> I got what I wanted!

> *Step 5:* DO
>> To get through this situation without yelling at Nathan. That would have only made me feel worse about it.

8. PARENTS OF CHILDREN WITH BEHAVIOR DISORDERS

Cheryl's success is similar to that of Susan. After several weeks of considering the hurtfulness of her thoughts and behaviors in many of the interactions with her son, Cheryl finally began to make changes in her thought patterns. This was all it took. The helpful thoughts that she had practiced generating in group on a weekly basis began to penetrate her thoughts in the situation as it was happening. Once she was able to think helpful thoughts, she found that helpful behaviors naturally flowed from them. As a result, her AO matched her DO. Just as in Susan's case, Cheryl continued to use the CSQ technique for the remainder of the group sessions.

OBSTACLES TO TREATMENT

Throughout the course of the 12 sessions, several obstacles were encountered that potentially limited the effectiveness of the treatment. Primary among the obstacles was attendance. Of the seven parents who attended the adult group each semester, only three to four attended on a regular basis. These three to four parents were those who achieved the maximal benefit from the group.

Another obstacle to treatment was resistance. Many of the parents expressed concern that it was not their behavior that needed to change but their children's behavior. They didn't understand how focusing on their thoughts and actions would help improve their children's behavior. In dealing with this resistance, we discussed two issues. The first was whether or not what they were doing was working for them. The response to this was a resounding no. Many of them tried one punishment after another without enforcing it consistently enough for it to be effective. Others were masters of consistency, but the behavior that they were consistently reinforcing was their child's bad behavior. For example, one parent would yell at her child every time he would do something annoying. This parent was inadvertently reinforcing the child's bad behavior with attention, albeit negative attention. Social learning principles were tied to these problematic behaviors to reiterate that both positive and negative attention are reinforcing to a child. As parents realized that past parental practices had not been effective, they became more willing to consider alternative strategies to behavior management.

In addition, the belief that parents have direct control over their children's behavior was challenged. The distinction between influencing their children's behavior and controlling it was made to identify a more logical point of intervention: parental thoughts and behaviors. Also, the importance of modeling the technique to their children was stressed as a major factor in facilitation of improved behavior. The importance of consistency was stressed throughout. For example, we focused on the importance of staying with one strategy. If parents consistently monitored their own thoughts and behaviors, they would not only be able to achieve personal outcomes that were desirable, but also they may inadvertently influence their child's behavior in the process. By becoming more consistent people, they became more consistent parents, and their children noticed.

The final obstacle in these groups is typical to any application of the CSQ. Initially, it is difficult to get the client to focus on realistic DOs. Consider the unsuccessful CSQs for both Susan and Gretchen and Cheryl and Nathan. In both cases, the mothers' DOs were related to their children acting differently. Our strategy was to go back through the CSQ and see whether there was anything they could have said or done to get their children to behave differently. In most cases, there were some actions that may have forced the children into obeying (e.g., spanking, yelling, threatening), but the parents were not pleased with these actions as options because they would not feel like good parents after they employed them. This process allowed the group to uncover alternative DOs, those that were more within the realm of the parents' control and thus more realistic. As in our two unsuccessful CSQ examples, these more controllable, realistic outcomes usually had something to do with the actions, feelings, or thoughts of the parent, not the child. It took several weeks to get the parents thinking of the interactions with their children in a self-focused way, but the results were promising. Not only did we see parents who were attentive to thinking and acting in a consistent manner with their children, but we saw the consistency generalize to other areas of the parents' lives. We saw parents interacting better with their spouses, with their parents, and with their colleagues. And, as often happens when patients begin thinking and behaving in a consistent, helpful manner, parents were able to shape or influence the behavior of those around them, including their children.

Our case studies illustrate the beneficial impact of CBASP when incorporated into existing manualized PMT treatments for use with parents of preadolescent boys and girls who exhibit externalizing behavior problems.

Although the evidence at this junction is anecdotal in nature, we believe that the inclusion of CBASP is supported theoretically. In the future, research pitting the combination of CBASP and PMT against PMT alone would help distinguish whether the inclusion of CBASP has any incremental validity in the treatment of childhood externalizing behaviors in terms of decreased parental resistance, increased treatment compliance, better identification of problematic behavior, and increased short- and long-term treatment effects.

Chapter 9

Children With Social Skills Deficits*

Social skills deficits are common among children with a variety of behavioral problems including Attention-Deficit/Hyperactivity Disorder, Oppositional Defiant Disorder, and Conduct Disorder. Children with these disorders often engage in negative behaviors that are intended to gain attention but that actually result in a lack of peer acceptance and, ultimately, peer rejection. This chapter demonstrates how the Cognitive Behavioral Analysis System of Psychotherapy can be modified for use with children, both in the individual therapeutic setting and in the group therapeutic setting. Two case examples provide support for the modification of the Cognitive Behavioral Analysis System of Psychotherapy, with particular emphasis on the analysis of the behavioral aspects of the treatment. However, consideration to children's own thoughts and feelings as well as the thoughts and feelings of others is also stressed in the modification of the technique.

In his book about children's social relationships, Asher (1990) describes some of the many functions of friends in childhood. He states that children's friends "serve as sources of companionship and recreation, share advice and valued possessions, serve as trusted confidants and critics, act as loyal allies and provide stability in times of stress or transition" (p. 3). Many children navigate their social world without difficulty, making and keeping friendships that are meaningful and fulfilling. However, some children find friend making tricky and often establish patterns of ineffective peer relationships. Problematic peer relations have been associated with a

---

*The primary authors contributing to this chapter were Karla K. Repper and Kimberly A. Driscoll.

variety of negative outcomes, including higher rates of delinquency, problems in school, and later psychopathology. Research has demonstrated that children with a variety of behavioral problems struggle significantly with peer relations, experience peer rejection, and, not surprisingly, display social skills deficits (McMahon & Wells, 1998).

Schaefer, Jacobsen, and Ghahramanlou (2000) define social skills as the ability to interact appropriately with peers in a given social context. Social skills include interactions that are acceptable, valued, and beneficial and include the abilities to communicate effectively, to demonstrate good sportsmanship, to resolve conflicts quickly, and to enter into conversations and groups with ease. Social skills likely contribute to social competence. Children who display social skills deficits in prosocial situations often resort to more severe conduct problem–related behaviors to gain attention (Slaby & Crowley, 1977), which can result in a lack of peer acceptance and, ultimately, peer rejection.

The *Diagnostic and Statistical Manual–Fourth Edition* (American Psychiatric Association, 1994) includes three disorders under the category of Attention Deficit Hyperactivity and Disruptive Behavior Disorders: Attention-Deficit/Hyperactivity Disorder (ADHD), Oppositional Defiant Disorder (ODD), and Conduct Disorder (CD). The prevalence rates for these disorders are 3%–5% in school-age children for ADHD, 2%–16% for ODD, and 6%–16% for boys and 2%–9% for girls for CD (American Psychiatric Association, 1994). Aggression, disruptiveness, and social skills deficits are essential features of these disorders; thus, it is interesting to note the lack of social skills training research with children diagnosed with ADHD, ODD, and CD.

Recently, social skills training programs have been developed in an effort to improve school-age children's social skills and to improve parent coping mechanisms when dealing with their children's behavior problems. Kaduson and Schaefer (2000) developed a 10-week social skills curriculum for parents and children that incorporates negative consequences, modeling, prompting, ignoring, and reprimanding into interesting lessons and homework assignments. The specific skills focus on conversational skills building, group entry, assertiveness, social problem solving, cooperation, complimenting, awareness of feelings, good sportsmanship, and smiling. Bloomquist (1996) developed a guidebook for providing skills training directly to parents, which addresses increasing parental involvement and positive reinforcement, changing parents' negative thoughts, enhancing positive family interaction skills, helping children to comply with requests,

9. CHILDREN WITH SOCIAL SKILLS DEFICITS
141

improving children's social behavior skills, and enhancing social and general problem-solving skills. Thus, in contrast to Kaduson and Schaefer's program, children are not actively incorporated into Bloomquist's training approach.

A CBASP TREATMENT APPROACH

The child therapy group at the Florida State University Psychology Clinic was held for 12 weeks. The skills outlined by Kaduson and Schaeffer (2000) were combined with the problem-solving approaches described by Bloomquist (1996) and McCullough (2000) (see Table 9.1 for a description of the skills taught). Two graduate student therapists co-led the children's group, which included five children. Two other graduate student therapists co-led the parent group. See Chapter 8 for a description of the parent therapy group, which was held simultaneously.

TABLE 9.1
Skills Taught in Group Therapy

Introducing yourself	Expressing your feelings
Beginning a conversation	Relaxing
Asking a question	Saying good-bye
Saying thank you	Dealing with group pressure
Ignoring distractions	Dealing with fear
Giving a compliment	Apologizing
Asking permission	Asking a favor
Being honest	Reacting to failure
Sharing	Dealing with losing
Joining in	Ending a conversation
Dealing with boredom	Deciding what caused a problem
Staying out of fights	Expressing affection
Problem solving	Accepting consequences
Dealing with anger	Negotiating
Dealing with another's anger	Smiling
Avoiding trouble	Having fun
Accepting consequences	Dealing with fear
Dealing with group pressure	Responding to teasing
Saying no	Accepting no
Knowing your feelings	Suggesting an activity

Note. From *Skillstreaming the elementary school child: New strategies and perspectives for teaching prosocial skills* (pp. iii–v) by Ellen McGinnis and Arnold P. Goldstein, 1997, Champaign, IL: Research Press. Copyright 1997 by Ellen McGinnis and Arnold P. Goldstein. Reprinted with permission.

The children who participated in the group presented with behavioral problems as reported by parents during an initial interview. Children with severe behavioral problems consistent with a diagnosis of CD, the most severe of the disruptive behavior disorders, were not included in the group. Instead, because of the nature of their behavior problems (e.g., cruelty to animals, fire setting), children whose symptoms were consistent with a diagnosis of CD were referred for individual therapy. The children in the group primarily had difficulties getting along with their peers and siblings, complying with parent and teacher requests, and acting in socially appropriate ways. Parents reported that their children behaved in annoying ways, had few friends, and failed to take responsibility for their actions.

FORMAT OF THE GROUP: INTEGRATION OF SPECIFIC SOCIAL SKILLS IN MODIFICATIONS OF CBASP

At the beginning of each group session, we introduced a new social skill, which was adapted from both Kaduson and Schaeffer's (2000) play therapy program and McGinnis and Goldstein's (1997) recommended strategies for teaching children prosocial skills. After the introduction, we conducted a short discussion about each of the components necessary for mastering the skill. For example, when we taught the skill joining a group, we discussed the four components of joining a group, which included making a decision about joining the group, deciding what to say, choosing a good time to join the group, and joining the group in a friendly way. Following introduction of the new skill, the cotherapists modeled the skill for the children using situations that they identified as problematic. Again, using the skill joining a group as an example, one cotherapist pretended to be playing basketball on the playground while the other cotherapist demonstrated how to join the game using the skill. Then, the children were provided with a hypothetical situation, and volunteers role played the use of the skill in the situation. Cotherapists not only provided feedback to the volunteers about their use of the skill but also solicited feedback from the other children. This provided an opportunity to teach and review the skill with the entire group.

Similar to the way in which we introduced, taught, and modeled individual social skills, we also instructed the children in the use of a seven-step Coping Survey Questionnaire (CSQ) based on approaches by McCullough

9. CHILDREN WITH SOCIAL SKILLS DEFICITS

(2000) and Bloomquist (1996). During sessions that focused on the CSQ, we reviewed the steps and asked group members to describe a problematic situation and then answer the following questions, given their particular problematic situation (Bloomquist, 1996):

1. What is the problem?
2. Who or what caused the problem?
3. What does each person think or feel?
4. What are some plans?
5. What is the best plan?
6. Did the plan work?
7. What could you have done differently to prevent the problem?

Step 1—What is the problem?—asks the children to state the problem simply and concisely and to limit the detail to descriptive information only. To do this, the children were encouraged to describe the situation as though it happened on a television program or a movie they had seen. The benefit of this step, as in the adult CSQ, is that the patient is forced to isolate problematic situations and to take an objective stance while describing it.

In Step 2—Who or what caused the problem?—the children must identify the source of conflict. Our group was focused primarily on interpersonal conflicts, and Step 2 encourages the children to focus on the roles they and others play in conflicts.

Step 3—What does each person think or feel?—asks the children to consider their own thoughts and feelings as well as the thoughts and feelings of others in an effort to promote sensitivity to the role of cognitive factors in achieving desired outcomes and to increase their awareness of how feelings of others can affect situations. For more advanced children, this step is sufficiently challenging to ensure sustained attention to the task.

Step 4—What are some plans?—asks the children to brainstorm what they could have done in the situation. Asking the children what they actually did in the situation and writing their behavior down as a plan provides an opportunity in the next step to evaluate their actual actions during the situation. This step offers a nonjudgmental way to examine actions insofar as the plan is treated the same as the potential plans offered by the children. Generally, three or four plans provide ample material for evaluation in the next step. This step provides the children an opportunity to creatively problem solve without emphasis on the right answer, and the therapist writes down all plans presented by the children, regardless of their viability or usefulness. The skills training component of the group helps the children to build a repertoire of social tools to plug in to this step of the CSQ, and we have found it helpful to encourage the children to consider these skills when generating plans during the initial training of the CSQ process. If the children present no appropriate behavioral plans, the therapist offers a brief suggestion, preferably a previously taught social skill, to include in the list of plans.

Step 5—What is the best plan?—requires the children to choose the best plan from the list of plans generated in Step 5. Doing this requires an evaluation of each of the possible plans. The cotherapists begin the evaluation of each plan by asking the children what might happen if each plan were enacted and to label the plan as helpful or hurtful based on the predicted outcome. While working with the children to evaluate the plans, the cotherapists ask the group leading questions in an effort guide the children to consider ways in which they could have used the previously learned social skills to prevent the original problem or to better the outcome of an already problematic situation.

Step 6—Did the plan work?—asks the children to consider specifically what they actually did in the situation and whether or not it worked out the way they wanted, as well as how their behavior was different from the best plan identified in the previous step. Although this step could be incorporated into Step 5, we feel it is important to pay specific attention to the actual behaviors of the children in the situation and to isolate them for evaluation. Positioning this step after Steps 4 and 5, which are usually fun and hopeful, reduces some of the potential stress, embarrassment, or anger felt by the children while evaluating their own behavior (and having it evaluated by others). Over time, it has been our experience that children habituate to this step and become increasingly better able to objectively analyze their behavior in relation to the outcome of the situation.

Finally, Step 7—What could you have done differently to prevent the problem?—asks the children to think about ways to prevent the problem altogether. Unlike the first six steps of our modified CSQ, which focus on handling a problem once it arises, this step focuses on making good decisions before a problem arises. Many children who have social problems struggle with impulsivity, and this step is designed, in part, to address this issue. However, it should be noted that there is little empirical evidence to suggest that psychosocial interventions are effective in reducing impulsivity.

9. CHILDREN WITH SOCIAL SKILLS DEFICITS

∽ CASE EXAMPLE 1 ∽

To illustrate the use of our modified CSQ in the group setting, we provide the following transcript of one child talking through a situation using the seven steps of the CSQ.

Simon is an 11-year-old boy who is in the fourth grade. He was tested for ADHD when he was in the first grade. Although he exhibited some of the symptoms of the disorder, a formal diagnosis was not made. Simon earns As and Bs in his classes and was placed in the gifted program.

Simon's mother described him as a know it all who acts as if he is an expert and often corrects people. In addition, he was described as argumentative and defiant. Simon reportedly denies all responsibility for his actions. Simon's teacher described him as an attention-seeking individual who often actually seeks negative attention. She also stated that Simon is immature at times and that he fancies himself a class clown. Simon's behavior resulted in placement on a behavioral program at school. In addition, he experiences peer rejection, which has resulted in Simon adopting a defensive/aggressive response style toward his peers and other authority figures. For example, when asked a neutral question by a peer or adult, Simon often assumes that he is being challenged and will respond accordingly with a sarcastic, caustic retort and occasionally will lash out physically.

Simon's behavioral symptoms were suggestive of ODD, although a formal diagnosis was not made. He clearly did not meet criteria for CD, and his mother reported that Simon did not exhibit any serious psychiatric symptoms, such as suicidal or homicidal ideations, hallucinations, delusions, or substance use. The following is a transcript of a therapist and Simon in a session.

Therapist: What is the problem?
Patient: I had to clean my room.
Therapist: Who or what caused the problem?
Simon: Well, what caused the problem is that there is this little car track called Nightmare Alley, and it was buried under all of this stuff and when I pulled it out from under the stuff, it all came flying out. There were several boxes, and it dumped everything on the floor.
Therapist: What does each person think or feel?

Simon:	Well, I was pretty upset because here I am standing in the middle of this huge mess up to my knees, and my mom was saying, "You've got to clean that up!" I guess my mom was mad, and there was all of this mess, and she thinks I just threw it out of the closet.
Therapist:	What are some plans?
Simon:	Clean it up. This probably wasn't the best plan, but I held off on cleaning it up for 3 or 4 days and that made my mom and dad really, really mad.

At this point the therapist states her confusion about who caused the problem. When she stated that Nightmare Alley car track caused the problem, Simon immediately stated, "Well, I caused the problem because I pulled it out and everything fell." The therapist then went back to the first step and clarified that Simon caused the problem by pulling the Nightmare Alley car track; the problem was not that he had to clean his room. Sometimes it is necessary to allow a child to complete a step incorrectly and take advantage of opportunities, such as in this example, for remediation and correction. Next, the therapist asked the group to get involved in this CSQ by providing ideas for plans.

Therapist:	Can anyone besides Simon think of a plan for this situation?
Group:	Clean it up. Delay cleaning for two more days. Just not clean it up at all.
Therapist:	Good. Simon, can you think of a skill we practiced earlier that would fit into this situation?
Simon:	I guess accepting consequences would work here.
Therapist:	How do you mean?
Simon:	Well, if I had accepted that pulling out Nightmare Alley and having all that stuff fall out would mean that I would have to clean my room, I might have done it right away rather than wait.
Therapist:	What about the plans of delaying cleaning for two days and just not cleaning up at all—what would happen if you did these?
Simon:	Well, I did wait for a few days, and that made Mom mad, and if I hadn't cleaned up at all, she would have been even madder!
Therapist:	OK, good. So tell me, what is the best plan?
Simon:	Accepting the consequences of pulling out Nightmare Alley and clean my room up right then.
Therapist:	(directed to the group) Do you guys agree with Simon that this is the best plan?
Group:	Yeah.

9. CHILDREN WITH SOCIAL SKILLS DEFICITS

Therapist: So did your plan work—not cleaning your room for a few days?
Simon: No—I got in trouble, and mom was mad.
Therapist: So what do you think you could have done differently to prevent this problem from happening?
Simon: If I had not pulled out Nightmare Alley from beneath the other toys, it would have prevented me from having to clean my room, from mom getting mad. Not pulling out Nightmare Alley would have been the best plan.

At this point the therapist suggests that not pulling out the Nightmare Alley car track would have been the best plan for Simon if he had been able to think ahead and guess that his other toys would fall down and make a mess. However, given that he did pull out the car track, she queried him about the best plan given the situation.

Simon: The best plan would have been to just clean it up and not wait.
Therapist: Good, Simon. I think you're getting the hang of it.

Simon quickly learned the format of the modified CSQ and the social skills that were taught. He demonstrated impressive use of the skills and modified CSQ in session, and he reported that on a few occasions he was able to use it proactively. For instance, he reported that he used the skill of negotiating one day at school when he and another child wanted to use the same computer game during free time. Simon reported that he remembered how to think about a situation and make plans, and then he remembered the skill of negotiating, which includes deciding what you want and whom to ask, talking in a nice voice to the person you want to ask, and offering something in return for what you want (McGuiness & Goldstein, 1997). Simon was able to use these steps to secure ample time with the desired computer game.

In addition to using our modified CSQ with the children in the group setting, therapists in our clinic have also been using it with individual child patients by incorporating it into the delivery of established or probably efficacious treatments of anxiety and depression.

CASE EXAMPLE 2

Anna is a 10-year-old girl who is in the fourth grade. Katherine, Anna's mother, brought her to the Florida State University Psychology

Clinic because of minor oppositional behaviors in the home and decreased academic performance at school. Anna's mother reported that Anna had become increasingly defiant over the past several months, and that the behavior problems began at approximately the same time that Katherine's boyfriend moved into the family home. Anna was reportedly defiant, and she frequently sought negative attention by annoying others and arguing. In addition, she repeatedly lied and denied responsibility for her actions. Anna was diagnosed with Disruptive Behavior Disorder Not Otherwise Specified because she did not meet full diagnostic criteria for Oppositional Defiant Disorder. Her mother reported that she did not exhibit any serious psychiatric symptoms, such as suicidal or homicidal ideations, hallucinations, delusions, or substance use. Katherine admitted that her parenting style was probably more permissive than the typical parent. She indicated that she was interested in fostering a close, friendshiplike relationship with Anna and found it difficult to discipline her. In contrast, Katherine's boyfriend demonstrated a more strict parenting style, demanding perfectionism and blind obedience. Katherine and her boyfriend could not agree on a parenting style that fit both of their needs.

The modified CSQ was used with Anna to decrease her lying and to increase the likelihood that she would take responsibility for her actions. The following is an example in which Anna accepted responsibility for her actions and successfully generated an appropriate alternative to the problematic behavior.

Therapist: So tell me Anna, what was the problem?
Anna: I got into trouble because I hit my cousin.
Therapist: Who or what caused the problem?
Anna: Well, my cousin caused part of it because she said something mean to me, but I guess I caused part of it because I hit her.
Therapist: What does each person think or feel?
Anna: My cousin feels hurt, and I feel bad about what I did.
Therapist: What are some plans?
Anna: I could say, "I'm sorry." I could have not hit her. I could not even worry about hitting her.
Therapist: Can you think of some skills we've talked about before that remind you of this situation?
Anna: Staying out of fights?
Therapist: Yeah—I think that's a good one here. Can you remember what the steps of this were?

9. CHILDREN WITH SOCIAL SKILLS DEFICITS 149

Anna: Um, I think they were stopping and counting to 10, deciding what the problem is, thinking about choices like walking away, talking to my cousin in a friendly way, and asking my mother for help.

Therapist: What do you suppose would have happened if you did that?

Anna: I probably would not have hit my cousin.

Therapist: So what do you think is the best plan?

Anna: Counting to 10 and don't hit her and walk away.

Therapist: What could you have done differently to prevent the problem?

Anna: I could have ignored what my cousin said to me and walked away so that I wouldn't have hit her.

Therapist: Good job, Anna, I think you picked a good plan.

Anna quickly learned the social skills and the format of the modified CSQ. At the end of each session, she was given several blank forms to complete as homework, and she usually completed them as instructed. On a few occasions she would fail to complete her homework; therefore, the CSQ would be completed in session. Anna clearly understood the format of the CSQ; however, she failed to use her skills proactively. Interestingly, it is likely that Anna chose not to use the skills she was learning for several reasons. One of the more likely reasons was Anna's desire for attention from her mother's boyfriend. By misbehaving, Anna was guaranteed attention from Katherine's boyfriend, albeit negative attention. Unfortunately, Katherine and Anna terminated therapy prematurely. Katherine and her boyfriend ended their relationship, and, according to Katherine, Anna's behavior improved dramatically once the boyfriend moved out of the family home.

OBSTACLES TO TREATMENT

The primary obstacle to treatment was the inconsistent attendance of our group members. The goal of treating children in group therapy is to provide an opportunity for the children to become acquainted with each other and to begin to form friendships within the groups that can then be used to practice skills and to receive feedback. In fact, as groups progress, children often begin to have conflicts within the group (mirroring their peer conflicts at school and in the neighborhood) that can provide opportunities for processlike interventions, which include putting group conflicts into a

CSQ. Small and inconsistent group attendance impedes the development of these relationships. In addition, poor attendance affects the key components required for success with the CSQ method. Learning and using the CSQ requires prolonged exposure to the method and subsequent practice and modification with a therapist.

Another obstacle to successful use of the CSQ is holding the children's interest with what is essentially a verbal method of analyzing situations. Occasionally our children reported that the CSQ was boring and indicated that they would rather play a game or engage in some other type of interactive activity. This is not surprising given that the children in our group often present with poor attention, hyperactivity, and impulsivity. Incorporating role plays in the reenactment of a situation provided an opportunity for the children to move around and be stimulated, while still allowing the steps of the CSQ to be practiced. We also find it crucial to maintaining group interest and engagement that all children participate in the generation of plans (Step 4) during a CSQ presentation by a group member.

In addition, we used a simple token economy in our group, where the children received tokens for participating and providing insight and had tokens taken away for rule-breaking behavior. The rules of the group were generated by the children at the start of the group and written on a board, which was displayed during each session. The rules included "Do Not Interrupt," "Be Polite," and "Talk in a Nice Voice," among others. Children who violated the steps of a previously taught skill during session were also subject to losing tokens. For example, after the skill beginning a conversation was taught, the group members were expected to make eye contact and talk in a normal tone of voice when addressing other group members and the cotherapists (both steps of this skill), and not doing both of these would result in a taking away of tokens. Likewise, successful completion of the steps of a skill would result in the earning of tokens. The prizes available to the children at the end of each session were directly related to the number of tokens earned during the session—more tokens meant better prizes. We found that this provided extra motivation for ongoing participation in the group activities—especially in the completion of CSQs.

Finally, the ultimate goal of McCullough's (2000) treatment is to train the patient to use the CSQ proactively. That is, the goal is to have the patients think about their desired outcome and how their behaviors and interpretations can influence the attainment of the specified outcome. Given the limitations in children's thinking and their inability to think ahead, combined with the impulsive tendencies that many of the children exhibited, few of the children reached the point at which they were able to use the CSQ proactively. Clearly, they were able to identify the consequences of their behaviors retrospectively, demonstrated by their competence in session with the use of the CSQ. Perhaps teaching the children's parents this modified CSQ and how to guide their children through it as well as encouraging families to facilitate ongoing CSQ practice at home would improve the likelihood that the children would master the CSQ process and implement it in their lives. In addition, when children have conflicts at home or school, parents could use the CSQ as a comfortable, neutral way of exploring the conflict with their children.

The integrated use of Situational Analysis using the CSQ format with prosocial skills training appears promising in the treatment of social problems in children with various symptoms of disruptive behavior disorders. Our experiences in both group and individual therapy settings suggest that children can be taught to use a modified CSQ in conjunction with specific social skills to examine problematic situations and to generate plans that would have helped them achieve a more desirable outcome. However, empirical examination of our claims must be conducted before therapists use our method as the sole treatment of children's peer rejection.

In addition to gauging the success of teaching an integrated CBASP/ social skills program by measuring the ability of children to use these methods in session, future attention should be given to other indicators of successful treatment. These other indicators may include the generalizability of the treatment to social situations in the children's lives, such as school, religious, or sports groups, and the decrease in conflict with peers as reported by the children and their parents and teachers. Additionally, measuring change in the children's severity of symptoms related to depression and anxiety prior to and following the conclusion of the treatment is critical to address the relevance of social skills improvement to mental health in children.

Social status improvement in children through targeted treatments is an area in which the research is, at best, mixed with respect to its effectiveness. Most studies that show improvements in the children treated with social skills training do so in very limited arenas. This is unfortunate because of the clearly demonstrated negative life implications (e.g., delinquency, aggression, depression and anxiety) for children who struggle to make and keep friends. Continuing to develop treatments that help children with poor peer relationships succeed in interacting with others and building meaningful friendships should remain a priority for clinical researchers invested in alleviating child psychopathology. We believe that this integrated approach to social skills training and situational analysis provides an incremental improvement to existing treatments and is deserving of empirical attention.

Chapter 10

Couples*

Treating couples in psychotherapy presents unique challenges, particularly because the couple is generally seeking treatment for relationship difficulties; however, these problems may be confounded by one, or both, partner's own psychopathology. This chapter provides a review of the available treatment approaches for distressed couples. Although the principles of the Cognitive Behavioral Analysis System of Psychotherapy are consistent with already available treatments, this chapter demonstrates the unique use of the treatment, in which couple distress is the primary focus and individual distress is addressed indirectly. A case example and transcripts are provided, along with an integrated discussion of the obstacles that may arise during treatment.

Working intensively with more than one patient simultaneously in therapy presents many challenges. Of course, treating a couple is unlike treating a patient, in that the therapist has to relate to the couple as a couple and as individuals, rather than just relating to one patient. Couples may present with a variety of problems, including lack of communication, trust issues, excessive arguments, infidelity, and financial issues. Unlike patients who seek therapy, couples are generally not given a specific diagnosis other than "partner relational problem." This category does little to describe the nature of the difficulty or the particular areas of concern. Working with couples can be challenging because the two individuals in the couple may have different goals in therapy, different levels of motivation, and strikingly different views about some issues. In addition, mood and anxiety disorders

---

*The primary authors contributing to this chapter were Kelly C. Cukrowicz and Jennifer A. Minnix.

153

on the part of one or both partners may complicate the relationship and may make working with the couple even more difficult. Though couples therapy presents unique challenges, there are techniques that seem to be useful in treating couple distress.

Four treatment approaches have shown varying levels of success with distressed couples, including Behavioral Marital Therapy (BMT), also known as Traditional Behavioral Couples Therapy (TBCT); Integrative Behavioral Couples Therapy (IBCT); Emotion-Focused Therapy (EFT); and Insight-Oriented Marital Therapy. BMT is by far the most widely evaluated treatment for couple distress (Baucom, Shoham, Mueser, Daiuto, & Stickle, 1998). This treatment involves teaching couples how to communicate and solve problems more effectively and helping couples to plan behavioral changes that increase the frequency of positive interactions. Based on many treatment outcome studies, BMT is considered an efficacious intervention specifically designed for treating distressed couples, though its long-term benefits are less clear (for a review, see Baucom et al., 1998). IBCT uses the principles of BMT but focuses more on acceptance of partner differences in an attempt to change not only behavior but also the emotional reaction to the behavior by the partner. Ideally, this intervention aims to reduce the stress that accompanies attempts by couples to change one another (Wheeler, Christensen, & Jacobson, 2001). Though not yet established as an efficacious treatment, preliminary studies suggest that IBCT is effective in reducing blaming while promoting positive emotional expression between partners, even when compared with BMT (Baucom et al., 1998; Wheeler et al., 2001).

EFT is an experiential treatment developed specifically within attachment theory that blends theoretical perspectives relating to the dynamics within relationships and acceptance of others' limitations (Greenberg & Johnson, 1988). This intervention emphasizes the centrality of emotion in marital distress and attempts to teach partners to communicate their emotional experiences and to meet their own attachment needs. EFT is considered an efficacious, though nonspecific treatment for couple distress (Baucom et al., 1998; Johnson & Lebow, 2000).

Insight-Oriented Marital Therapy offers couples interpretations that allow them to understand their own incongruent beliefs, maladaptive relationship rules, and developmental issues (Johnson & Lebow, 2000). This treatment has shown promising posttest and 4-year follow-up results in treating distressed couples and is considered to be probably efficacious (Baucom et al., 1998; Johnson & Lebow, 2000). Many of the issues addressed in the interventions currently used to treat distressed couples, such as highlighting problematic emotions and behaviors, are consistent with those emphasized in the Cognitive Behavioral Analysis System of Psychotherapy (CBASP).

CBASP works to help patients recognize the connection between what they think and what they do and the consequences of both. Without this connection, the environmental domain has no power to influence a patient's behavior because the patient is failing to respond appropriately to important cues. This connection allows patients to deal more effectively with life stressors, interpersonal relations, and environmental demands. Though this method of psychotherapy has shown very clear promise with depressed patients (Keller et al., 2000), its use has never been systematically studied with populations of couples. However, the underlying goals of this treatment approach may prove useful in teaching couples to interact with each other and the environment in a manner that gets them what they want.

CBASP first teaches patients to identify ways in which they contribute to their own personal living dilemma. Once the patient understands the types of thoughts and behaviors that keep the patient from getting what he or she wants, a choice can be made to live life differently. In essence, this treatment approach focuses a patient's attention on the consequences that he or she elicits from the environment. In the case of couples, this approach may highlight thoughts and behaviors that contribute to the distress that these patients are feeling within their relationships. In addition, it might be useful in highlighting the goals of each partner of the couple and the degree to which they are congruent. This treatment approach can provide a patient with insight into the consequences of his or her own behavior. Using this approach with couples, one patient may gain insight into his or her own thoughts and behaviors as well as those of the other partner. Once these connections have been highlighted, the couple has the means and ability to make specific changes that may lead to greater satisfaction with the relationship.

MODIFICATION OF CBASP FOR COUPLES THERAPY

The first stage of couples therapy is assessment of the problem areas. This includes a detailed picture of the problem areas, factors that serve to increase or decrease distress associated with these problems, resources that each partner brings to the relationship (e.g., good problem-solving skills), exacerbating factors that each partner brings to the relationship (e.g., Axis I or II disorder, violence), onset of the problems, Desired Outcome (DO) of each partner for the various problem areas, and level of commitment to the relationship. It is recommended that the Dyadic Adjustment Scale (Spanier, 1976) or the Marital Satisfaction Inventory (Snyder, 1979) be administered prior to the first interview to obtain preliminary information pertaining to several of these areas.

Following the assessment of the overall functioning and problem areas for the couple, the therapist provides the couple with feedback illustrating the conceptualization of their relationship. This should include both the problem areas and the areas of strength. It is important that the therapist then allow the couple an opportunity to respond to and express their feelings about this conceptualization. This may also provide the therapist with valuable information as to whether the couple will be invested in continuing with treatment.

The second stage of CBASP implementation for couples is to describe the treatment model in a way that is easily understood. This description should clearly illustrate the components of the Coping Survey Questionnaire (CSQ) and how this method of evaluating problems will bring the couple closer to resolution. Specifically, this method helps the couple to recognize maladaptive patterns of interaction and the ways in which these patterns can be resolved. The following is an example of this type of description:

> We are going to be working together in the next few months in an effort to solve some of the problems that have developed in your relationship. The core principle of this treatment is the discrepancy between what you want to happen in a specific situation and what is actually happening. By examining the patterns of interaction between the two of you, we will begin to uncover ways in which you can both get what you want. How does that sound?
>
> Specifically, I will ask each of you to complete a Coping Survey Questionnaire, which we call CSQs, about an interaction that occurs between the two of you. In our session, we will talk about the situation, what each of you were independently thinking during the situation, what each of you did during the situation, what each of you wanted (we call that the Desired Outcome), and what each of you actually got (we call that the Actual Outcome) from the situation. Using this method will allow us to determine ways in which your thoughts and behaviors are interfering with your ability to get your desired outcome.

10. COUPLES 157

After the couple has a general understanding of the therapy, the therapist should discuss the couple's commitment to the treatment. First, the couple should agree to attend an hour-long session each week for at least 12 weeks. This is the minimum amount of time typically necessary for lasting change to occur in psychotherapy. It is important to stress that the components of the treatment must be fully mastered before permanent change can occur. Premature termination is likely to result in less than optimal outcomes for the couple (e.g., return to previous maladaptive methods of relating to each other and coping with disagreements). Second, it is also crucial to obtain a commitment that each partner will be an active participant in the treatment. Often, one partner is less invested in improving the relationship than the other. If this is the case, this partner needs to make a decision about his or her commitment to the therapy process prior to the implementation of this treatment. The treatment will be less effective if one partner does not commit to active participation. Third, it is also important that the couple agrees to independently complete CSQs each week. If a couple does not understand the need to complete these independently, it is necessary to explain to them that they will almost always have different thoughts and behaviors, as well as different DOs in a situation, and it is necessary to know what each of them independently brings to these interactions. Fourth, the need for cooperation should be stressed because it is possible that one partner will dominate the other, which may consist of interrupting the other partner, dominating the conversation, or speaking for the other partner. When this happens, the therapist should inform the couple that in their sessions each partner will have a turn and that each partner will not be permitted to speak while the other is speaking.

USING THE CSQ WITH COUPLES

In the next phase of therapy, the primary goal is to teach the couple to individually complete the CSQ and to illustrate how this method leads to change. Begin by asking each person to describe a situation of conflict that occurred within the last few days (Step 1). Ask each partner to fill out a description of the situation on his or her own CSQ. Then ask each partner to write his or her interpretations of the situation (Step 2). Next, ask the partners to record their behaviors or what they did or said in the situation (Step 3). The next step is to ask each partner to record the Actual Outcome

(AO; Step 4). Finally, ask each partner to record the DO, that is, what he or she wanted out of the situation (Step 5).

After the partners have completed their own CSQ, review the CSQs independently. Ask each partner to read what he or she wrote for each of the five steps. It is helpful to emphasize each step as Step 1, Step 2, and so on to establish a common way of describing each step of the CSQ. Once each partner's CSQ has been summarized, it is helpful to highlight similarities and disparities between the two. This is an important factor in the resolution of conflict for the couple. The partners individually rate whether their interpretations helped them or hurt them in obtaining their DOs, and it is important to link each thought to the DO. When interpretations prevent a partner from getting his or her DO, request alternatives that would have helped. Ask for descriptions of how the alternatives would have helped the partner to get his or her DO. Finally, ask each partner if he or she had done all the helpful alternatives, would the DO have been attained? Repeat this process for the step involving behaviors for each partner of the couple.

At this point, it is necessary to focus on the DO that each partner chose. First, determine whether each partner recorded a DO that is compatible with, or the same as, the other partner's DO. In cases where the DOs conflict, it is important to discuss the reasons for this. Was the situation ambiguous? Is there a communication problem? Do they just want different things? Ask the couple how they feel about these differences or similarities. When disparate DOs cause a tremendous amount of distress, the couple may feel motivated to try and communicate their DOs so that they are both striving for a common goal. The therapist should ask the two partners to think of a compromise DO that they can both agree on and to generate several interpretations and behaviors that would help to achieve the compromise DO. In some situations, each partner records a DO that is the same or complementary to his or her partner's DO. At this point, it should be obvious which interpretations and behaviors impeded the attainment of the DO. Highlight these for the couple so that they will have a greater understanding of the things they can change to achieve these DOs.

Once a couple has mastered the steps of the CSQ, it is necessary to teach the partners to generalize it beyond the specific situations discussed in therapy sessions. This can be accomplished by asking questions such as "How can you use this information about changing your thoughts and behaviors to get what you want in other situations?" "Are there other areas of conflict in your relationship?" and "Do you have trouble in other rela-

10. COUPLES 159

tionships or with your children? If so, let's think about how you can apply the things you have learned to those situations and relationships." At this point the therapist should consider having the couple complete a prospective CSQ about one of these situations, in which they are asked to consider what a future situation might be and what the DO will be. Completing the interpretations and behaviors section in a way that maximizes their chances of success illustrates to the partners how the CSQ can be used proactively to reduce the likelihood of future conflict.

⟶ Case Example ⟵

Lisa and Greg were married for 3 years and had been experiencing relationship difficulties for 1.5 years. They dated the 2 years prior to their marriage. Greg's goals for therapy included clarifying his and Lisa's personal identities and determining whether they should continue their marital relationship. He wanted Lisa to stand up for herself and express her opinions freely. Lisa wanted to remain married to Greg and to improve their communication. She was frustrated that Greg failed to recognize her contribution to the family. The couple felt that they both attempt to please each other in overly accommodating ways that undermine their needs. Though they reported some happiness in the relationship, they also reported engaging in frequent unresolved arguments that left both of them feeling upset. Greg felt encroached upon by Lisa, whereas Lisa felt that Greg was distant. In addition, Lisa was experiencing symptoms of depression and anxiety, including mood swings and social isolation. The following describes a situation explored during their eighth therapy session. At this point in therapy, they were very familiar with the CSQ method.

Therapist: It's nice to see the two of you again. Did you bring in a CSQ that we can go over together?

Greg: Yes, but I always go first. Maybe Lisa can start this time.

Therapist: That seems reasonable. Greg, I'm sure I don't have to remind you, but try to hold your comments until Lisa has finished going through her version. Lisa, are you ready? Why don't we start with Step 1, a short description of what happened.

Lisa: Well, what happened is that Greg came home from work, and he was in a bad mood. I guess he was tired or something. Anyway, he was grumbling about dinner, but I had already decided not to cook because I thought we could go out for a change. I spent most of the day cleaning the house, and I did not feel like cooking dinner. He told me he was hungry and tired and wished there was something ready for dinner.

Therapist: Okay, on to Step 2. What did the situation mean to you?

Lisa: Well, I thought that I should have just cooked something because I knew better than to plan on going out without asking Greg first. I also thought that he does not even appreciate how nice the house looks or how hard I worked all day. I assumed he was angry with me for not being considerate of the fact that he had a hard day and that he was tired, which made me feel guilty. I immediately apologized for not being a good wife and started pulling things out to cook a quick dinner. I made it clear that I was upset by my tone of voice and almost started crying.

Therapist: Great. You also covered Step 3 by describing your behaviors. We can go on to Steps 4 and 5. What was the outcome of the situation and what did you want the outcome to be?

Lisa: Greg became frustrated that I was upset, and we got in an argument. He did not even understand what was wrong with me. We ended up ordering a pizza and ignoring each other for most of the evening. What I wanted was to greet him when he arrived and go out for a nice dinner. I also wanted some acknowledgment of the work I did around the house. It was a huge mess when he left for work. I thought we could both relax after a long day and then go home and watch a movie or something. I certainly did not get what I wanted in this situation.

Therapist: Thanks, Lisa. Greg, back to Step 1. It is your turn to tell us your version of the story.

Greg: Okay. Well, I walked in from work, and Lisa was watching TV on the couch. There was nothing in the kitchen for dinner like there usually is, so I asked Lisa what we were having. She got all upset and started apologizing and crying. I had no idea what she was so upset about. After we ordered pizza, she told me that she had wanted to go out, but whatever. That's when we got in the argument.

Therapist: Let's move on to Step 2. So what were your interpretations?

Greg: I thought that she was all upset again for no reason. When I figured out she wanted to go to dinner, I could not understand why she did not just tell me that's what she wanted—I'm not a mind reader. I thought that I did not need her starting a fight with me after such a long day. So I ordered a pizza and then sat on the couch to watch TV. I did not say much to her for the rest

10. COUPLES

of the night. I was in a bad mood when I got home, and my tone of voice may have been a little rough, but I wasn't upset with her at first.

Therapist: Okay, you've covered Step 3 by describing what you did in the situation. We can move on to Steps 4 and 5. So what was your DO for this situation? Did you get what you wanted?

Greg: I just wanted to come home from work, have something to eat, and take it easy for the rest of the night. We could have gone out to eat or stayed in, I did not really care. Instead, I came home, got into yet another argument with my wife, and went to sleep bitter and frustrated. So no, I did not get what I wanted at all.

Therapist: Okay, you both did a great job. Clearly you two have this method down pretty well. I noticed that both of you wanted to spend a relaxing evening together. Often, you two have very different DOs. This might make the resolution a little bit easier. What I also heard is that Lisa wanted you to appreciate the work she did around the house, Greg, and you wanted her to tell you what she had planned for dinner, whether it was at home or going out.

Greg: Yes, she never tells me what she wants. She just gets upset, and I have no idea why. I wouldn't have minded going out, I just didn't know she wanted to.

Lisa: Well, you were so grumpy that I thought you were mad at me for not having dinner laid out on the table the minute you walked through the door. You don't even care that I cleaned all day even though you were complaining about what a wreck the house was.

Therapist: Clearly both of you are still feeling frustrated with the way this turned out. I'd like to go back through these CSQs and see if we can come up with some alternate interpretations for this situation. This time we'll start with you, Greg.

Greg: All right.

Therapist: You wanted to come home, have dinner with your wife, and settle in for the night, correct?

Greg: Yes, but I also wanted her to just tell me what she wanted to do for dinner, instead of getting her feelings hurt for no reason.

Therapist: Maybe we should take a closer look at your interpretations. You said that you thought that she was upset again for no reason. Did that help you or hurt you in terms of getting what you wanted?

Greg: Well, I guess it hurt me because I automatically assumed she was being ridiculous and that just made me angry.

Therapist:	Can you think of another interpretation that might have helped you get what you wanted?
Greg:	I could have thought that she was upset and probably had a reason for that, so I should try to see what's wrong. That would have helped me because I would not have gotten as angry and maybe we could have talked calmly about things rather than get in an argument.
Therapist:	Great. Now let's move on to your second interpretation. You said that you didn't need her starting a fight with you for no reason. Did this interpretation help you or hurt you?
Greg:	This one definitely hurt me because, again, I just assumed she was being unreasonable and that I had not contributed to the situation at all. I was being selfish because I was grumpy about my bad day. I guess if I had thought that maybe I had hurt her feelings, I would have been more in tune to my own behavior and we might have avoided the argument.
Therapist:	You are doing a great job coming up with these alternatives, Greg. Next, you said that your tone of voice wasn't very pleasant when you got home. Is that right?
Greg:	Yeah, and I can see what you're getting at. I guess that hurt me because it might have made her think that I was angry with her. Maybe I should have made it clear that I wasn't upset with her right when I got home, instead of snapping at her.
Therapist:	Good. You also said that you just ordered a pizza and then ignored her for most of the night.
Greg:	Yes, and that hurt me because it hurt her feelings even more and just prolonged the argument. If I had just not been so stubborn and talked to her about it, we might have solved it within the first few minutes I was home instead of ruining the whole night.
Therapist:	Would changing this behavior have also helped you achieve your other DO, which was for her to tell you what she wanted?
Greg:	Hmm, well, maybe it would have helped, but I guess ultimately that depends on her. I guess that may not be the best DO.
Therapist:	Though I understand that you want her to feel comfortable telling you what she wants, it may be an unrealistic goal for you because it relies on her behavior, which you can't control. Can you think of a related but more appropriate DO?
Greg:	I guess I would want to not take out my own bad mood on her, which might make it easier for her to tell me what she wants.
Therapist:	I like this one and I can see how the alternatives you came up with might help you achieve this.
Greg:	Yeah, maybe.
Therapist:	Okay, Lisa, let's move on to your CSQ. In this situation, you

10. COUPLES

Therapist: wanted to go out to dinner with Greg and then spend a nice evening together. You also said that you wanted him to acknowledge your work around the house. Is this right?

Lisa: Yes, pretty much.

Therapist: Your first interpretation was that you should have known better than to plan to go out without asking Greg. Did this thought help you or hurt in terms of getting what you want?

Lisa: Well, maybe it hurt me because it made me feel like I had to ask permission from him instead of just telling him that I would like to go out to dinner. I guess a better interpretation would have been to think that he was clearly tired from a long day, but maybe he would enjoy a casual dinner out somewhere.

Therapist: That sounds good. Your second interpretation was to assume that he was angry with you. Did this help or hurt?

Lisa: Well, this one definitely hurt because my feelings were hurt when I thought he was angry. If I had just thought that maybe he had a bad day and his mood had nothing to do with me, I wouldn't have gotten so upset.

Therapist: Great. Your third thought was that he did not even care about the work you had put into cleaning the house. Does that sound about right?

Lisa: Yes. This one hurt because, again, it just hurt my feelings and upset me. I should have thought that he just walked in the door and probably hasn't had a chance to even notice the house yet. Then I would not have been upset, and maybe he would not have gotten frustrated. Then we could have maybe had a nicer night together.

Therapist: Will this new interpretation help you with your second DO, which was for him to acknowledge your work around the house?

Lisa: Well, maybe. But I can't really make him say anything no matter what I do, so maybe it's not a very good DO.

Therapist: Absolutely right. You can't control someone else's behavior. Can you think of an alternate DO?

Lisa: I guess that one of my DOs might be to not get so emotional over things because I know that it often leads us to big arguments.

Therapist: Great. It seems that these new interpretations might help you with that outcome. Do you agree?

Lisa: Yes, if I can actually do it.

Therapist: You said that you immediately apologized to him for not being a good wife and scrambled to find something for dinner, is this right?

Lisa: Yes, and I know that what I did wasn't helpful because it only made him angry with me since he had no idea why I was upset.

	I should have just told him that I was sorry he had a bad day and that I wanted to go out for dinner.
Therapist:	You also said that your tone of voice and the fact that you were almost crying were the ways you showed him you were upset. Did this help or hurt?
Lisa:	This hurt because he often ignores me when I act like this. I should have just talked to him about what I was feeling. Maybe then we could have resolved things much faster.
Therapist:	You two have both done an excellent job. Now that we've gone through both of these CSQs, what kinds of thoughts do you two have?
Lisa:	It seems that we are both making assumptions about the other instead of just talking. It seems to get us both in trouble.
Greg:	I agree, and I also feel that we are so used to fighting with each other that we expect negative reactions and emotions from each other. But, really, we both just want to spend some relaxing time together.
Therapist:	Was talking through this situation helpful?
Greg:	Yes, it allows me to see how I contributed to the argument, rather than just blaming it on her.
Lisa:	It was helpful for me because I realize that being submissive actually seems to hurt our relationship, even though I feel like I'm doing it so we won't fight so much. It's sort of ironic.
Therapist:	Do you think that the things you learned today might apply to other situations?
Greg:	Sure. It makes me more aware of how I come across to her. I need to be more mindful of how I express to her that I'm in a bad mood without hurting her feelings. Maybe then she will feel more comfortable asserting herself with me.
Lisa:	I also realize that if I just told Greg what was really on my mind more often, we would probably get along much better.
Therapist:	Well, we've blazed through this session. We'll continue to analyze these problem situations and generalize them to other areas of your lives. You two are doing a great job so far.

OBSTACLES TO TREATMENT

Patients often have difficulty mastering the steps of the CSQ. If generating interpretations proves difficult, ask questions such as "Fill in the blank for me. This situation meant blank to me." If generating interpretations continues to be difficult, it may be necessary to provide possible interpretations that someone might have in that type of situation. If either partner has difficulty generating behaviors, the therapist may provide prompts, such as "If I were a fly on the wall, what would I have seen each of you doing in this situation? What did you say? How did you say it? What was your body language? What was your facial expression? Did your body language communicate an attitude or frustration?" If either partner continues to have difficulty with this, provide possible examples of behaviors someone might express in a similar situation. In some situations it will not be obvious what went wrong. Often couples say they had all the right interpretations and did all the right things to get their DOs. At this point, it is necessary to look at the DOs to determine if one or both are unrealistic.

The couple may not have established adequate communication or problem-solving skills to achieve their DOs or each of them may have a DO that relies on the actions of the other. In the former case, focus the couple on the need for small steps toward improvement rather than all-at-once change. If communication has been hindered, the couple will need to repair this a little at a time. The therapist may want to include additional homework assignments geared toward these areas of skills deficit. When a couple is aiming toward DOs that are unrealistic, ask them to think of more realistic DOs. When each partner in a couple generates a DO that relies on the other partner of the couple, it is crucial to illustrate how these outcomes can be problematic. Each patient is only responsible for his or her own behavior; he or she cannot fully control the behavior of the other partner. Encourage the couple to generate alternative DOs for the situation that are not tied to the actions of partners.

This chapter presented an adaptation of the CBASP method for couples therapy. This treatment approach has only recently been applied to couples. Differences in DOs, as well as problematic thoughts and behaviors that partners of a couple have that are interfering with their happiness, are highlighted. There are several advantages for the use of this treatment. First, this method can be used by each partner of the couple to improve other problematic areas. Specifically, this treatment method can be used to target symptoms of Axis I disorders, such as Major Depressive Disorder (McCullough, 2000), which has been demonstrated to cause problems in marital relationships. Another advantage of this treatment is its broad applicability to relationships. The CBASP method can be used to target other problematic relationships with children, co-workers, friends, and others. Though this method seems to be a promising new advance in couples therapy, no randomized studies have been conducted to determine its efficacy in this particular mode of therapy. Future research should be conducted to compare this treatment to the other forms of couples therapy.

PART IV

Other Issues and Groups

Chapter **11**

.

Anger Management Problems*

Although it is not an independently diagnosable condition, excessive or uncontrolled anger constitutes a critical feature of many adult and childhood psychiatric disorders and can significantly interfere with several domains of life functioning. This chapter explores the phenomenon of anger and briefly summarizes existing anger management techniques. The comparative use of the Cognitive Behavioral Analysis System of Psychotherapy is highlighted by its attention to the cognitive, emotional, and behavioral experience of anger; its straightforward integration of relaxation; and its inherently nonconfrontational approach that makes it particularly amenable to clients prone to anger. The versatile application of CBASP for anger management is illustrated in group format at a residential juvenile detention facility, and by a case description of its use in an outpatient university clinic.

The problem of excessive or uncontrolled anger is unique among the areas of intervention discussed in this book in that it is not independently diagnosable. However, it is a problem that is pervasive across the diagnostic axes of the *Diagnostic and Statistical Manual of Mental Disorders* (*DSM*; American Psychiatric Association, 1994), as well as across differences in gender, age, and culture. Insufficient anger control can manifest in childhood disorders such as Conduct Disorder (e.g., bullying, threatening, fighting, intimidating), and in Oppositional Defiant Disorder (e.g., frequently losing one's temper, arguing with adults, being angry and resent-

---

*The primary authors contributing to this chapter were Andrea B. Burns and Bradley A. White.

ful; American Psychiatric Association, 1994). In adults, insufficient anger control functions as a diagnostic criterion for Antisocial Personality Disorder (e.g., irritability and aggressiveness, including repeated physical fights or assaults), Borderline Personality Disorder, and for the rare diagnosis of Intermittent Explosive Disorder, characterized by extreme aggressive outbursts (American Psychiatric Association, 1994). Beyond its diagnostic implications, excessive anger may have far-reaching consequences for multiple areas of functioning, including job performance, marital satisfaction, maintenance of friendships, and effective parenting. As such, the effective treatment of inappropriate anger is a matter of great clinical importance.

WHAT IS ANGER?

The phenomenon of anger is multifaceted in cognitive, emotional, physiological, and behavioral components. As such a complex entity, it has been conceptualized within the framework of nearly every conceivable approach to the study of mental health, from cognitive behavioral to psychodynamic (e.g., Leifer, 1999; Ornstein, 1999; Robins & Novaco, 1999). Regardless of the perspective, there are commonalities to the understanding of anger that make it one of the basic human emotions recognizable and identifiable across cultures. Anger is characterized by physiological events, such as a pounding heart, a rise in blood pressure, a rush of adrenaline, increased muscle tension, and a flush in the cheeks (e.g., Deffenbacher, 1999; Mayne & Ambrose, 1999). Of course, these physiological conditions might also characterize love, anxiety, excitement, and a host of other emotions. In addition to such qualities, then, anger bears a purely emotional component distinctly negative in tone, along with a cognitive component laden with thoughts such as "I want to hit him," "How dare she do that to me?" or "That's just not fair!" When combined, these cognitive, emotional, and physiological features may lead to the behavioral components of anger, such as physical or verbal violence, impulsivity, and damage to property.

EXISTING TREATMENTS OF ANGER

Like sadness, euphoria, and fear, anger is a natural emotion experienced by all people at times. As such, it is not inherently problematic but may

11. ANGER MANAGEMENT

become so when the experience of anger exceeds what is normal in the population and when it interferes with a person's daily functioning. This may occur when the individual is easily and frequently provoked to anger, when the individual copes with that experience of anger in dangerous or destructive ways, or when both of these situations occur simultaneously. As such, a variety of therapeutic treatments have been developed to address this problem.

There are multiple theoretical vantage points from which to approach the treatment of anger, but by far the most frequently empirically studied has been the cognitive behavioral approach. Although there have been too few studies conducted to indicate any overall superiority of this approach to the treatment of anger (Gerzina & Drummond, 2000; Mayne & Ambrose, 1999), the efficacy of this treatment modality has been repeatedly demonstrated in various populations, including adolescent psychiatric patients (Snyder, Kymissis, & Kessler, 1999), children (Sukhodolsky, Solomon, & Perine, 2000), college students (Deffenbacher, Dahlen, Lynch, Morris, & Gowensmith, 2000) and adults (Gerzina & Drummond, 2000).

WHAT CBASP HAS TO OFFER

The methods available for the treatment of anger within a cognitive behavioral approach may include a multitude of elements, either alone or in combination (Deffenbacher, 1999). Such methods may aim to enhance the individual's awareness of his or her anger symptoms through activities such as self-monitoring exercises and role plays. Alternately, one could intervene between the event precipitating anger and the response to that event through methods such as cool-off time. Relaxation training aims to modify physiological reactivity, whereas cognitive interventions focus on identifying and altering maladaptive thought processes. Communication and assertiveness skills could be taught and practiced to help the patients attain more productive methods of meeting their needs.

With so many cognitive behavioral tools already available in the clinician's repertoire, what is the value of adding the Cognitive Behavioral Analysis System of Psychotherapy (CBASP)? In short, the particular process and methods of CBASP provide an exceptionally efficient and useful framework within which to present the concepts emphasized in any type of cognitive behavioral therapy (CBT). This method addresses in one simple, five-step process the cognitive, behavioral, and emotional components of the patient's experience of anger and can easily be combined with other treatments more directly emphasizing the physiological aspects of anger. The process is relatively easy to learn and is brief enough to conduct within the constraints of a 50-min therapy session. Moreover, CBASP is equally applicable in an individual or group format, resulting in maximum use for the practicing clinician.

Beyond its utilitarian value, the philosophy and structure of CBASP conveys to patients that therapy will take on their bigger anger problems one situation at a time, rather than attempting to change them all at once. Patients can have confidence that with each situation that goes well, the encompassing problem is gradually but steadily chipped away. This breaks therapy into digestible chunks for the patient, making the notion of change less sweeping, and thus less alarming, in its scope.

Finally, the specific approach of CBASP is unique in its nonconfrontational approach to the treatment of anger. The role of the therapist is not to challenge the patient or to label the patient's thoughts or behaviors as maladaptive or distorted but rather to simply guide the patient through a series of steps that arrive at a simple question: "Did you get what you wanted out of this situation?" The patient comes to his or her own conclusions regarding this issue and determines the helpful or hurtful nature of each of his or her interpretations and behaviors in relation to the achievement of a specified goal. In doing so, the patient becomes the initiator of change in therapy. The therapist is accordingly freed from the burdens of directly challenging or confronting the patient and assuming the responsibility for correcting the patient's thoughts and actions. The therapist's ability to serve a collaborative role in this manner could contribute invaluably to the therapeutic alliance and to patients' motivation for and compliance with therapy.

ADAPTATION OF CBASP TO THE TREATMENT OF ANGER: INDIVIDUAL THERAPY FORMAT

Preliminary Interventions

Whether applied to an individual or a group format, the basic structure of CBASP is readily modified and applied to the treatment of excessive anger. Under both circumstances, the overall system outlined on the Coping Survey Questionnaire (CSQ) may be maintained and applied to situations provided by the patients, as described in more detail later.

However, it may be beneficial to include an additional component to treatment designed to address directly the physiological component of anger not typically tapped by the CSQ. Patients presenting with anger control problems may continue to be angry or may experience a resurgence of anger in therapy when recalling the situations that previously elicited an anger response. Accordingly, the therapist may wish to include a relaxation component in the therapy to help the patient step back and attain sufficient composure to cognitively explore the situation. A variety of relaxation techniques may prove useful in this endeavor, including Progressive Muscle Relaxation (PMR) and guided meditation. Patients may also be encouraged to generate their own suggestions of techniques that work for them, such as exercise, listening to music, or journaling.

Step 1: Generating Situations

Patients will likely have little trouble coming up with example situations to which the method may be applied in Step 1 because problems with anger control almost invariably yield an array of interpersonal difficulties. The only limitations on acceptable situations for analysis are that they are discrete, specific (as applies to the use of CBASP for any problem), and related to the patient's difficulty with anger management.

Step 2: Interpretations

In Step 2, the patient must identify his or her interpretations of the situation at the time the situation occurred. It must be noted that patients who demonstrate difficulty with impulse control, including impulsive anger, may have difficulty recognizing the existence of a thought process at times when they get angry, believing instead that they are not thinking at all or that they simply "snap." We shall return to this matter and discuss it in more depth later, in conjunction with other obstacles to treatment. However, once patients are shown how to recognize their thoughts in the situation, certain patterns are likely to emerge consistently, including thoughts of entitlement (e.g., "I want it, so I should have it"), blaming (e.g., "He's making me act this way"), mind reading (e.g., "She wants to hurt me"), and magnifying (e.g., "He's always picking on me—I can't stand it!"). Over the course of therapy, patients may be encouraged to note how their specific thoughts in the situations they encounter may map onto these more global ways of thinking. However, CBASP differs from traditional CBT in its emphasis on evaluating thought patterns in terms of their impact on attainment of Desired Outcomes (DOs), rather than on the type of logical errors and distortions they may represent.

Additional Step: Feelings

Because the experience of anger tends to be visceral, we recommend the inclusion of an additional step in the CSQ process, following the exploration of the patient's cognitions and preceding the itemization of the patient's behaviors. This additional stage focuses the patient's attention on objectively examining his or her feelings within the situation, in response to interpretations the patient had during the event. Without question, anger is likely to be the primary feeling noted in the situations presented, and this is appropriate considering the goals of treatment. However, for individuals with anger control difficulties, an angry reaction to an event may also mask feelings of sadness, hurt, or anxiety (Paivio, 1999). Asking patients to identify their emotions at this stage in the process is intended to make clearer the notion that their anger does not come "out of the blue" but rather follows from their interpretations during the event. Although this sequence of event-cognition-emotion may be explicitly taught to the patient in traditional cognitive therapy, in CBASP the patient's understanding of this process is allowed to emerge on its own, as the patient becomes more adept at using the CSQ.

Step 3: Behaviors

Following this slight deviation from the typical sequence of steps on the CSQ, in Step 3, the patient is asked to detail his or her behaviors within the selected situation. The patient should specify not only the *what* but also the *how* of his or her actions, including gestures, posture, facial expression, and tone and volume of voice. Patients with anger problems often have difficulty communicating their wishes in a nonaggressive, assertive, verbal fashion; thus, nonverbal aspects of communication may serve a dominant functional, albeit dysfunctional, role. Patients who have trouble describing their behaviors can be encouraged to reenact for the therapist exactly what they did and how they did it. It is necessary to include these details to paint the richest possible picture of the event as it took place. Therefore, the patient should be encouraged to provide three to four of his or her specific behaviors in the situation so that the therapist (and other group members, if applicable) can develop a clear and comprehensive image of the situation as it actually transpired.

Step 4: Actual Outcome

Following the patient's specification of the situation, interpretations, feelings, and behaviors, it is appropriate to proceed to Step 4 in the CSQ sequence: the Actual Outcome (AO). Patients may prefer to view this step as describing the consequences of their behavior—the natural result of whatever action they chose to take. In addition, the AO may be viewed as the next precipitating negative event in an ongoing cycle of escalating anger, similar to the negative spiral of depression conceptualized by Mc-Cullough (2000). Patients with anger control problems are likely to have experienced multiple situations that escalated from a relatively minor incident into a major, possibly violent outburst. By viewing the CSQ steps in a cyclic fashion, patients will likely understand how the AO of one situation may become the triggering event for a second or third situation, with its concomitant sequence of interpretations, feelings, and behaviors. In such cases, it can be beneficial to complete several CSQs (time permitting) to help the patient identify each pass through the cycle.

Step 5: Desired Outcome

In the CBASP method in general, and in the treatment of anger in particular, defining the DO is the lynchpin of the therapeutic process, which occurs in Step 5. Encouraging a patient to develop internal motivation to change his or her behavior necessitates a sustained focus on how the patient might more effectively obtain desired rewards and avoid punishment or undesired situational outcomes. Although patients may be able to perceive that they are unhappy with the pattern of behaviors, or that these behaviors are leading to interpersonal, financial, or legal problems (including court-ordered therapy, as in our case study), without a clear criterion for evaluating their thoughts and behavior in a given situation, it may be impossible for patients to identify exactly what they are doing wrong or how to change to achieve their goals. The DO furnishes this point of comparison, by forcing patients to become goal oriented and to evaluate their own behavior in light of the established goal.

One critical adjustment may be needed at this stage to accommodate the specific demands of the patient with anger problems. In the typical process of CBASP, the DO is meant to be the patient's goal *at the time,* within the selected situation. It is on the basis of this goal that the interpretations and behaviors listed in the previous steps are to be evaluated in terms of their helpful or hurtful nature. However, DOs of patients presenting with insufficient anger control, in the moment, might involve inappropriate or excessive expressions of anger (e.g., beat up another person, put the boss in her place, take out one's feelings on the family car). In such cases, it may become clear during the analysis phase of the process that the individual did get what he or she wanted in the immediate sense, in that the reported DO and AO matched (e.g., the patient did beat up another person). DOs involving strong or uncontrolled expressions of anger may actually serve a desired function in the short term, but, within the scope of the situation (e.g., by releasing stress, communicating frustration, achieving goals by intimidation), they typically conflict with the patient's long-term goals (e.g., avoiding legal problems, making a marriage work, succeeding at a job) and often create the very problems that led the patient to therapy. In such instances, as is always the case in CBASP, the therapist should resist the urge to challenge the patient's DO directly or push the patient to conceive of a "better" DO. Rather, the therapist should allow the CBASP process to illuminate for patients the concurrence of their short-term DO and the AO and acknowledge that the outcome of the situation was immediately satisfying for the patients. The therapist may then encourage patients to consider their long-term goals as well as short-term goals and to generate a second, alternative DO on the basis of more long-term objectives. If both types of DOs can be generated by patients, the remainder of the CBASP process may reveal the discrepancy between these sets of objectives and allow patients to maintain a focus on their reasons for pursuing treatment: the attainment of long-term goals.

Once the DO has been specified, the therapist poses the simple question: "Did you get what you wanted?" The answer to this question may appear to the therapist to be so obvious that it is tempting to delete this question. However, this impulse should be resisted and the question posed nonetheless to make absolutely clear to the patient—with a verbalization from the patient—that the DO was not obtained. It is at this moment that the potential distinction between short- (i.e., anger-driven) and long-term DOs may become critical because patients with an anger-based DO may indicate that in some respects they got what they wanted (e.g., wanted to beat someone up and did), but in other respects they did not get what they wanted (e.g., lost a job because of fighting). Again, in such cases, it is entirely acceptable for the therapist to acknowledge the possibility of some goals being met while others were not. Through the analysis of numerous problematic situations over the course of therapy, it will ultimately become clear to patients that although immediate impulses (i.e., short-term, anger-

11. ANGER MANAGEMENT 177

driven DOs) are consistently being gratified by their current cognitive and behavioral approach to situations, their larger, more important long-term goals are not being reached. The therapist can trust in the CSQ process to bring this distinction to light rather than attempting to force patients to acknowledge it.

In the event that the AO matches the patient's DO (and this outcome was not anger based but based on long-term goals), there is cause for celebration. It should be stressed to the patients that success situations are every bit as worthy of attention and analysis as failures because patients benefit as much from focusing on what went right as on what went wrong, for use in future situations. Early in therapy, however, it is far more likely that in the majority of situations provided by the patient, the AO and DO will be discrepant (particularly with respect to DOs based on long-term goals).

Remediation

Once the patient recognizes this disparity, the therapist may proceed to the remediation phase of the treatment. In this phase of CBASP, the patient revisits each of the interpretations and each of the behaviors itemized in Steps 2 and 3, respectively, and for each one poses the question, "Did that thought or behavior help me or hurt me in attaining my DO?" Having established the goal for the situation, the patient must evaluate each interpretation and behavior with respect to that goal. Here, again, the possibility of multiple, conflicting DOs may be a factor. In the event that the patient has specified two distinct DOs, two distinct remedial passes through the CSQ would be indicated so that the patient might evaluate each interpretation and behavior with respect to a single goal. It is recommended that the entire remedial phase be completed regarding one DO before shifting attention to the second so that the patient may separately consider each interpretation and behavior with respect to each goal. By repeatedly engaging in this process over the course of treatment, patients can discover that the very same cognitions and behaviors that help them to achieve short-term, anger-driven goals may interfere with the attainment of long-term goals without the therapist having to explicitly teach this concept.

As with typical CBASP procedure, it is recommended that attention first be devoted to the patients' interpretations, followed by their behaviors during the remediation phase, to maintain the structure of the first pass through the CSQ. The therapist's role is to help patients clarify and explain their answer to the "helpful or hurtful" question, while leaving the judgment of helpfulness or hurtfulness to the patient. To this end, the therapist may pose the follow-up question: "How was that helpful or hurtful?" The goal of such a follow-up probe is not to expose flaws in the patient's logic but simply to understand the reasoning behind the patient's evaluation of that thought or action. It may well be the case that an interpretation considered hurtful by the therapist might be viewed in a different, more helpful way by the patient, and the therapist should remain open to this possibility. In general, however, patients have relatively little difficulty perceiving the impact of their interpretations and behaviors on their DOs.

It may be noted that we have not advocated a similar analysis of the helpful or hurtful nature of the patient's reported feelings in the remediation phase, although an explication of the emotional component of the situation was advised earlier. This omission was deliberate because to evaluate an emotion in such a way is to imply that it might be directly revised in the future, independent of modifying interpretations and actions, a suggestion we deem untenable. We have argued for a discussion of the patient's feelings within the chosen situation as a route to clarifying for the patient the sequential manner in which emotions, such as anger, arise out of cognitive interpretations and how anger is related to (and sometimes masks) other emotions. However, in the remediation phase, the emphasis is on the patient's cognitions and behaviors alone because these elements are more easily revised, with the understanding that a shift in emotion should follow naturally.

Once the patient has labeled each interpretation and behavior as helpful or hurtful with respect to the DO, direct remediation takes place. For every interpretation or behavior identified by the patient as hurtful, the therapist inquires, "What could you have thought or done instead that would have been more helpful in attaining your desired outcome?" The patient is thus encouraged to make his or her own revisions to the scenario, reforming it into an event in which the patient would have been more likely to attain the specified DO. When alternatives are constructed, the therapist may further question the patient as to how the new interpretation or behavior would have improved the odds of attaining the DO. Early in treatment, it is likely that the patient will have difficulty imagining realistic alternative interpretations or behaviors that might have been applied to the situation. Should this difficulty arise, the therapist may focus the patient back on the DO by using various questioning methods to lead the patient to some possibilities or by suggesting some possibilities for the patient to consider. As treatment progresses, the patient should become more adept at generating such alternatives independently. By the end of the second pass through the CSQ, the patient has revised each hurtful interpretation and behavior into a helpful one, which could increase the likelihood of achieving the DO.

Again, as noted previously, in the event that during the first pass through the CSQ the patient found that he or she did achieve the DO (particularly if this outcome was positive and contributed to long-term goals), the remediation phase should not be bypassed. Although such events are causes for celebration, they are also opportunities to reflect on how the patient's interpretations and behaviors in that situation resulted in his or her attainment of a goal.

ADAPTATION OF CBASP TO THE TREATMENT OF ANGER: GROUP THERAPY FORMAT

The previous discussion focused on the manner in which CBASP might be conducted with individual therapy patients. However, the method is easily transferred to a group environment. In such a situation, the differences include one significant modification to the process—patients' taking turns providing situations—and the potential for group input and feedback. Although patients need to take turns providing situations for analysis, other group members might contribute and thus benefit substantially. For example, they might help the focal group member to elaborate and clarify each step of the CSQ, to generate revisions for the thoughts and behaviors identified, and to determine whether his or her interpretations and actions were helpful or hurtful, in light of the expressed DO. The therapist leading such a group must take care to encourage a nonjudgmental stance among group members to maintain the collaborative spirit of the therapy. Throughout the course of the group, patients should be encouraged to complete CSQs between group sessions so that even when they are not called on to share in group, the process is nonetheless being practiced regularly, and progress is being monitored by group leaders.

We have implemented such a group format of CBASP for anger management at a high-risk secure detention and rehabilitation facility run by the Department of Juvenile Justice in Florida. The facility houses approximately 250 adolescent boys convicted of felony crimes, most of whom have numerous charges on record and have failed attempts at rehabilitation in less restrictive settings. Those who display ongoing or pervasive anger-related behavioral problems are required to complete an anger management group, consisting of 12 weekly sessions. At the start of group, patients are provided with a Daily Hassle Log, in which they record two hassle situations each day in a simplified CSQ format. At the start of the session each week, two of the members are asked to share one log entry each in a discussion. Cotherapists moderate the discussion, encourage active group participation, and visually chart on a dry-erase board the process of the elaboration and remediation of the CSQ steps.

With few exceptions, the boys with whom we worked at this facility tended to show a reduction of acting-out behaviors following participation in therapy, although some required additional time to warm up to the therapeutic process. Furthermore, although no data are currently available on the impact of group CBASP anger management treatment on residents' aggressive or otherwise angry behavior following release, the staff members at this facility anecdotally attest to the dramatic behavioral improvement on campus since the institution of this treatment program.

It should be noted that on either an individual or a group basis, patients of CBASP for anger management may be children or preadolescents or inmates of a correctional facility, as described previously. Although many of the principles presented in this chapter readily translate to such populations, other special aspects of child and correctional therapy must be taken into account as well. The reader is directed to Chapter 9 of this book, which specifically addresses the use of CBASP with children, and to Chapter 12, which addresses CBASP in correctional settings.

CASE EXAMPLE

To more clearly illustrate the application of this particular technique to the treatment of anger, we present below a case study of an adult patient in individual therapy at the Florida State University Psychology Clinic, an outpatient treatment facility serving the Tallahassee, Florida, community.

Sheldon is a 25-year-old man, employed part-time as an office manager. He was ordered by the court to attend 12 sessions of anger management treatment after he was charged with domestic battery for pushing his girlfriend to the ground during a domestic dispute. During the intake session, Sheldon acknowledged a history of diffi-

11. ANGER MANAGEMENT

culty with emotional expression and anger control and indicated that he was highly motivated to overcome these problems and to learn to cope better with interpersonal confrontations. Based on objective personality test results and information provided at intake, Sheldon was given a *DSM–IV* diagnosis of Impulse-Control Disorder Not Otherwise Specified.

The nature of anger and the general cognitive-behavioral model were presented in the first session. Because Sheldon had difficulty identifying and verbally expressing his level of anger in given situations, an anger vocabulary was developed, using Sheldon's terms, to permit a working dialog between him and the therapist. For instance, Sheldon identified a low level of anger (1 on a scale of 1–10) as *bothered*, whereas 4 out of 10 was *ticked off*, 7 was *angry*, and 10 was *furious*. Sheldon then constructed an anger hierarchy by identifying several situations, which he had previously experienced, that corresponded to these various levels of anger. The antecedents and outcomes of these situations were explored briefly in the second session to introduce Sheldon to CBASP and to examine the causal chain between interpretations, feelings, actions, and consequences. (Although not critical to the successful application of CBASP with all patients with anger problems, the therapist is encouraged to consider whether similar exercises may benefit particular patients.)

Sheldon also was given a packet of CSQ forms and instructed to complete two or three CSQs a week on any significant events in which he experienced some anger, with the modification that he indicate the level of anger experienced in relation to his interpretations (herein is the interjection of the feelings component omitted in standard CBASP). The following is a transcript from the third therapy session, in which a Situational Analysis (SA) was elicited from Sheldon in CSQ format regarding an event that had occurred since the previous session:

> *Step 1:* Describe what happened:
>> I was resting, watching TV all morning because I didn't have to work. My girlfriend came in the living room and asked, "Can we go out and do something fun for a change?" I asked her some questions, then she called her mom and said she's coming home because she's "too young to be cramped up in this house." I lied back down. A little while later she calmed down and said, "I want to go out to eat now." So we went out to eat.

It is noteworthy that, unlike some patients when first learning CBASP for anger management, Sheldon was fairly adept at keeping interpretations out of his description of the situation.

> *Step 2:* Describe your interpretation(s) of what happened:
> "What is she thinking? Is she testing me?"
> "What does she expect? We're both trying to pay our bills."
> "She has an upper hand over my life; I don't have control."
> "There's nowhere to go anyway because my cousin is out of town."

This step took some time because Sheldon was reluctant to acknowledge having interpretations that, upon reflection, he feared made him look like a mean person. The therapist intervened in two ways, first by asking Sheldon whether labeling himself as "mean" or "bad" might be an overgeneralization because nobody does only bad or only good things. Sheldon concurred. The therapist then asked, "More important, is worrying about how you look in my eyes helpful to our mutual DO of completing a CSQ?" Sheldon agreed that it was not and then revealed the aforementioned interpretations.

> *Anger level:*
> "6 out of 10. I was pretty upset."

> *Step 3:* Describe what you did during the situation:
> I said loudly, "There's nothing to do! What is there to do? There's nothing in this town but clubs and movies, just like you told your friend the other day! What do you want from me?"

Sheldon was reluctant to describe his tone of voice, gestures, facial expressions, and posture. The therapist decided to try to overcome this defensiveness by humorously exaggerating what one might have done: "Did you jump up, get all in her face like this, and yell 'There's nothing to do!'?" Sheldon chuckled and replied:

> When I said it, I probably had a confused and mad look. I just shrugged and kind of threw my hands up in the air. Then I lied down on the sofa again and looked away from her and stared at the TV.

> *Step 4:* Describe how the event came out for you (AO):
> "She wasn't angry anymore as far as I could tell, and we went to eat, but I didn't want to go because I was still upset."

11. ANGER MANAGEMENT

Step 5: Describe how you wanted the event to come out for you (DO):

Initially, Sheldon proposed three DOs:

> I wanted her to not be angry with me for watching TV.
> I wanted to know what she wanted to do.
> I wanted to rest, watch TV, and relax.

He was reminded that it is helpful to identify (if possible) a single realistic and attainable DO; thus, he revised his DO accordingly:

> I wanted to know if there was something I could do later that would make her happy, while still getting to watch TV and relax.

Sheldon was then asked whether or not he had achieved this corrected DO, to which he responded, appropriately, "No." As noted earlier, sometimes patients specify angry, hostile, or aggressive behavior as the immediate DO. Because none of Sheldon's DOs included such behavior, the discussion of a separate DO based on long-term objectives was not necessary.

During the remediation phase, Sheldon was able to specifically identify how his interpretations and actions had probably interfered with various aspects of his DO. He spontaneously noted:

> As far as my interpretations, I guess I could have thought, "There's always something we can go out and do. Not everything costs money. Maybe she just feels neglected and wants to spend time together." . . . I should have just asked her calmly what she would like to do and whether it could wait for another hour while I enjoy the game I was watching.

Sheldon conceded when the therapist asked whether these modifications would have helped him achieve his DO, remarking "probably all of it." The therapist commended Sheldon for his progress in analyzing the situation and developing more productive alternatives to try out in similar situations.

OUTCOME OF CBASP FOR SHELDON

Sheldon successfully fulfilled the requirements of his court-ordered anger management therapy and elected to continue therapy for several additional sessions to continue to work on communication and assertiveness issues. He and his girlfriend decided to separate, and Sheldon's subsequent DOs focused on making this as smooth a transition as possible. Though he admitted being mildly frustrated that he would not likely receive the money he felt she owed him, he intended to maintain peaceable relations with her for the sake of his relationship with their daughter. During his time in therapy, Sheldon required no further interventions by the police.

In the sessions prior to termination, Sheldon displayed moderate insight into the nature of his problems and seemed to be coping much more effectively with anger and frustration. He made strong progress in session with identifying interpretations and behaviors that had previously interfered with his DOs with his girlfriend. Additionally, he presented a number of events later in his therapy that suggested that he had internalized the structure and process of the CSQ and was able to use its methods effectively.

OBSTACLES TO TREATMENT

Even when the general process of CBASP is tailored to the treatment of excessive anger in the manner outlined previously, certain obstacles to treatment may remain.

Identifying Cognitions

One of the main difficulties encountered with patients whose behavior is characterized by impulsivity is their frequent difficulty recognizing the existence of a thought process between an event and a behavioral reaction. Patients frequently describe themselves as "snapping" or "losing it," as though a fundamental loss of control takes place in which thought plays no role. Such a belief may originate from the misconception that if one were thinking, one would not do anything so impulsive or destructive as patients with anger control problems sometimes do. This is where a review of the cyclical pattern of escalating anger may prove useful, by helping the patient to see that an emotion as strong as anger does not emerge from nowhere. A salient example such as the following may help to drive this point home: "You are waiting in line at the movies, and someone bumps into you from behind. You nearly fall over." Many patients, on the basis of this information, would claim that their reaction would be an angry one.

However, add an element to the situation, such as, "You turn around and see an elderly blind woman standing there," and patients will admit that they would not be so angry. When questioned as to what makes the difference, patients generally see that in the first instance they assumed they were pushed intentionally—a hostile interpretation—whereas in the second scenario they were provided with an alternative interpretation—the women was blind and did not know where she was going. Illustrative examples such as this one may help patients to understand that although they may be lightning quick, thoughts do indeed occur before emotion flares, and if the thoughts change as they did in the example, emotional change should follow.

Therapeutic Alliance and Investment in Treatment

The philosophy and method of CBASP are largely conducive to a positive therapeutic alliance, by encouraging a collaborative relationship between therapist and patient. However, the therapist must be prepared for the possibility that the excessively angry patient may be unwilling to engage in therapy (i.e., not completing homework assignments, not working at applying new ideas generated in session). This is particularly likely to be the case with court-ordered or incarcerated patients. Such patients may be participants in therapy not because of a desire to change or a dissatisfaction with their lives but because of a legal obligation. Moreover, such patients may have some incentive to present themselves as either more or less impaired by their anger control difficulties than they are in actuality, depending on the specifics of their legal predicaments. There is no fail-safe solution to these pitfalls of therapy, particularly when patients fail to fully participate in the completion of homework assignments. However, to the extent that the therapist can engage the patient in the process, the inherent supportive, collaborative, nonjudgmental stance of CBASP provides the optimal circumstances under which trust in the therapist's ability and desire to help may be recognized. Ultimately, it is the patients who make the decision as to whether they are getting what they want out of specific situations encountered, and, in the likely event that they are not, the therapist is in a position to provide some tools for improving that condition—a proposition that is hard to reject out of hand.

Frustration With Progress

Although the CSQ process is inherently simple and straightforward, it can be arduous for the patient, who may have difficulty believing that the revisions conducted after the fact with the CSQ may ever be applicable in real time. Patients with anger control problems are often impulsive and suffer low frustration tolerance, becoming easily discouraged by slow progress, setbacks, or relapse ("I know this stuff, but I can't seem to do it when I need to!") The therapist's role is to assure the patient that the recognition and evaluation of his or her own thoughts and behaviors is like any other skill—one that initially requires a great deal of attention and energy but that ultimately becomes second nature through extensive rehearsal and practice in real situations. While the patient works to develop these skills, the therapist can encourage him or her to look for ways in which the specific interpretations and behaviors delineated in the chosen situation might generalize to other similar situations so that the patient might begin to see connections and patterns in the events of his or her daily life.

Excessive and undercontrolled anger is a component of numerous clinical diagnoses and a contributor to impairment of basic life functioning for many individuals, making the effective treatment of anger a matter of great clinical import. Although there is no clear empirical consensus about whether or not a superior method of treatment exists, the recent psychological literature contains numerous sources of support for the contention that a cognitive behavioral approach to therapy is effective and can result in the reduction of both self-reported anger symptoms and angry and aggressive behaviors as rated by others. The incremental value of the treatment method proposed in this chapter is its ability, in one succinct five-step process, to address the cognitive, emotional, and behavioral components of the experience of anger, as well as its ease of combination with methods designed to address the physiological components of anger (e.g., relaxation training). In a collaborative and judgment-free system, the therapist helps the patient to determine, in the context of discrete situations, how to manage anger and increase success at achieving his or her goals. This process is easily adapted to serve patients of all ages, using either an individual or group format, and fits easily within the constraints of a time-limited session. Clearly, research is needed to ascertain the true effectiveness of this treatment modality, but in the absence of such conclusive evidence, the potential application of this process to the problem of anger management remains nonetheless persuasive.

Chapter 12

Correctional Settings*

> The use of the Cognitive Behavioral Analysis System of Psychotherapy is certainly not restricted to the outpatient clinic; rather, it may be effectively applied within the confines of the correctional setting. This chapter describes the interpersonal, emotional, and behavioral problems often encountered by prison inmates and forensic hospital inpatients and demonstrates, via session transcripts, how the Cognitive Behavioral Analysis System of Psychotherapy may be effectively applied to address the issues unique to incarcerated populations. A brief discussion of potential barriers to the implementation of mental health treatment in general, and the Cognitive Behavioral Analysis System of Psychotherapy in particular, within correctional settings is also provided.

Few would disagree that incarceration qualifies as a significant stressor that requires a good deal of emotional and behavioral adjustment for successful adaptation. An incarcerated individual, who might have never experienced a great degree of stability or structure in the past, is suddenly forced to live according to strictly enforced sets of rules and regulations. Correctional environments are settings in which certain authorities control even trivial life events, such as when and where one can sleep, eat, talk, and walk. Incarceration also represents a separation from loved ones; a loss of social support, liberty, security, acceptance by society, and material possessions; and, in most cases, the removal of the opportunity for opposite-gender sexual relations. It can serve as a major financial burden to both the confined individual and the family left behind. In short, correctional facilities are environments rife with stress and stressful situa-

---

*The primary authors contributing to this chapter were Lorraine R. Reitzel and Sarah A. Shultz.

tions, requiring a great deal of adaptability, coping, and resilience on the part of their inhabitants.

If severe enough, adjustment problems can lead to an Adjustment Disorder diagnosis. An Adjustment Disorder in correctional settings is a failure to achieve the level of coping and resiliency required for a successful transition or adaptation to the demands of the environment. *The Diagnostic and Statistical Manual of Mental Disorders–Fourth Edition* (*DSM–IV*; American Psychiatric Association, 1994) defines Adjustment Disorder as a period of time in which an individual experiences significant personal distress above and beyond what is expected or in which social, occupational, or behavioral functioning is disrupted, within 3 months following the commencement of a particular stressor. Estimates of prevalence in the general population range from 5% to 20% (American Psychiatric Association, 1994). In the *DSM–IV,* Adjustment Disorders are specified by their major symptom expressions and include the following: with Depressed Mood, with Anxiety, with Mixed Anxiety and Depressed Mood, with Disturbance of Conduct, with Mixed Disturbance of Emotions and Conduct, and Unspecified (American Psychiatric Association, 1994). The treating therapist must be sure that symptomatology does not meet "criteria for another specific Axis I disorder (e.g., a specific Anxiety or Mood Disorder) or is [not] merely an exacerbation of a preexisting Axis I or Axis II disorder" (American Psychiatric Association, 1994, p. 623). Instead, symptoms must be a reaction to a particular stressor, which in correctional settings is usually, although not always, a reaction to some or all aspects of confinement. This disorder can be acute (resolved within 6 months of onset) or chronic (with symptomatology lasting beyond 6 months) in nature. Most Adjustment Disorders in correctional settings are chronic because the particular stressor (e.g., transition to prison life) does not cease until the individual is released from confinement, which is many times longer than 6 months from their entrance into the system. Compared with other settings and other stressors prefacing adjustment difficulty, Adjustment Disorders in correctional settings warrant special attention given the high rate of chronicity, suggestive of the relative severity and seriousness of the disorder in these settings.

For many individuals, the adjustment from free life to a life of confinement is difficult. Problems with adjustment are quite common in correctional settings. In a recent national survey of 830 correctional psychologists, Boothby and Clements (2000) found that 20% rated adjustment issues as one of the primary four areas of psychological problems that they

12. CORRECTIONAL SETTINGS

encountered and treated in practice. Only depression, anger, psychoses, and anxiety were rated as more common areas of intervention (Boothby & Clements, 2000). The importance of exploring an appropriate and effective treatment for adjustment problems in prison and forensic hospitals is clear given their frequency in these settings.

As mentioned previously, the presenting symptomatology of adjustment problems can vary from patient to patient. However, due to the particular nature of correctional environments, behavioral indicators of difficulty with adjustment are somewhat predictable. In some sense, the presentation of adjustment problems in correctional settings can be either passive or active in nature, based on the coping and adjustment styles of the patient.[1]

PASSIVE-TYPE ADJUSTMENT PROBLEMS

The individual exhibiting passive-type adjustment problems is likely to come to the attention of mental health staff by self-referral or perhaps by the referral of custodial staff. The patient may be within a year or so of initial confinement and adjusting poorly, as evidenced by sad mood, difficulty falling asleep or sleeping excessively, and weight change. The patient may engage in excessive rumination about outside contacts and afford little attention to developing any inside contacts or relationships with other inmates or patients. The patient may attempt to procure specialized sleeping quarters, such as those that house primarily older individuals or those that have a low patient to room ratio. The patient may make excessive requests to see medical staff for general malaise or aches and pains. The patient may also come to the attention of staff following an attempt of self-harm. Alternatively, the patient might be a target for financial or sexual victimization. As a result of victimization or fear of victimization, a prison inmate, for example, might request protective custody (i.e., voluntary

---

[1] Although the depiction of adjustment problem types is based solely on the experience of the chapter's first author in working with male prison inmates, there are no extant reasons to believe that the descriptions are not applicable to women as well. Although the following portrayals may capture a majority of the behavioral symptoms, it should be noted that the presentation of adjustment problems or an Adjustment Disorder can take many forms. The profiles described do not, and do not attempt to, comprehensively represent all forms of the diagnosis, nor do all the symptoms described need to be present to make such a diagnosis.

placement on segregation so that he or she may have a personal cell and a higher degree of staff supervision) or seek a transfer to a different housing unit or facility. In a prison setting, the patient might eat alone in the dining hall or avoid large congregations of inmates by purchasing the majority of his or her food from the canteen. The patient may have had some difficulty coping with problems prior to incarceration (e.g., substance abuse) but lacks a significant history of past mental health intervention. Thus, the patient is likely to report that the onset of symptoms as described previously began at arrest or incarceration.

If symptoms are severe enough, patients with passive-type adjustment problems are likely to meet diagnostic criteria for Adjustment Disorder with Depressed Mood, Anxious Mood, Mixed Anxiety and Depression, or Unspecified, depending on the actual symptom constellation. Adjustment Disorder with Depressed Mood may resemble a mild form of depression, marked by withdrawal from others, crying spells, and sad mood. The patient exhibiting Adjustment Disorder with Anxious Mood may display clinical symptoms of anxiety not meeting criteria for another major disorder, such as generalized worry, tension, or paniclike symptoms. The patient with Adjustment Disorder with Mixed Anxiety and Depression, as the name implies, shows some combination of the two. Finally, the patient with Unspecified Adjustment Disorder may present with unverified somatic ailments or with "social withdrawal, or work or academic inhibition" (American Psychiatric Association, 1994, p. 624).

ACTIVE-TYPE ADJUSTMENT PROBLEMS

The individual exhibiting active-type adjustment problems is most likely to come to the attention of mental health staff by custodial referral following rule-breaking behavior, although self-referral is possible as well. Though most of the time the patient can get along with staff, the patient may expect special treatment on occasion and tends not to react well when limits are imposed. The patient might act aggressively with peers as well and may fare especially poorly in a correctional setting due to nonviolent or violent rule violations, resulting in a high rate of, for example, infractions and placements in segregation. As a result, these patients may come to the attention of correctional clinicians fairly quickly due to their acting out and the potential security hazards their actions present. These patients may be within a year or so of confinement and not appear to accept that they need to adjust old behavioral patterns to adapt well to the new environment. For some, this might be due to long-standing antisocial personality traits that are not easily amenable to accommodation based on environmental changes. Many of these patients meet criteria for a diagnosis of Adjustment Disorder with Disturbance of Conduct or with Mixed Disturbance of Emotions and Conduct. The latter diagnosis would obviously be appropriate for a case in which emotional symptoms (e.g., sad mood, anxiety) were cooccurring with the inappropriate, aggressive, or otherwise antisocial behaviors.

It should be noted that although these descriptions are couched in the context of difficulty with the process of initial adjustment to confinement, this symptomatology is not limited to the period following initial incarceration. Adjustment difficulty can emerge, for example, following a transfer from one prison to another, such as when one is demoted from a less-secure to a more-secure environment, or it may also emerge when an inmate is given a lengthy segregation term to complete. In the latter case, what few freedoms inmates had with regard to movement and activities are removed and inmates can be isolated in a cell for up to 23 hr a day, leaving only 1 hr for brief monitored showers and exercise alone in a small, secured area. The segregation units of prisons are rarely empty, and at times prisoners are released into the general population with only a fraction of their rule-violation time served to make room for a new offender. However, segregation sentences of 3 months or longer are not uncommon in some prisons and may result in difficulty with adjustment as evidenced by conduct problems (e.g., loud and consistent banging, feces smearing and throwing) or emotional problems (e.g., withdrawal, crying spells, refusal to leave cell).

Adjustment problems in correctional settings may also emerge for reasons not directly related to confinement. For example, patients might have difficulty adjusting to a medical condition, such as HIV or hepatitis, diagnosed during their stay in prison or in the forensic hospital. The transmission of these conditions is not uncommon in correctional settings due to sexual activity among patients or the sharing of tattoo needles. Patients might also have difficulty adjusting to the loss of something outside the correctional setting, such as the reduction or loss of social or financial support due to a divorce or a death in the family. Moreover, as patients might not automatically be granted permission to leave prison or hospital grounds to attend funeral services in the case of a death in the family, the inability to see the deceased one last time or to grieve with the family members may result in significant difficulty adjusting to the loss.

Finally, mental health conditions existing prior to confinement can further compromise or complicate adjustment to correctional settings. By way of example, Antisocial Personality Disorder (ASPD) is an Axis II disorder common in correctional settings. In fact, whereas estimates of the prevalence of ASPD in the general population range from 1% to 3% in women and men, respectively, the prevalence rates have been found to reach 30% in some clinical settings and may exceed that number within prison and forensic settings (American Psychiatric Association, 1994). Gacono, Nieberding, Owen, Rubel, and Bodholdt (2001), for example, reported an ASPD base rate of 45% to 75% in forensic settings. ASPD is characterized by "a pervasive pattern of disregard for and violation of the rights of others" (American Psychiatric Association, 1994, pp. 649–650) and is marked by failure to conform to social norms, deceitfulness, irritability, aggressiveness, disregard for the safety of self and others, and lack of remorse. By its very characterization, ASPD suggests a negative adjustment to an environment where one is required to live and work closely with others, especially when such an environment demands conformance to norms and enforces this demand via 24-hr supervision of behavior. ASPD can negatively affect adjustment to correctional settings by leading the inmate to respond to externally imposed structure and rules by acting out (as in an active-type adjustment problem, described previously).

TREATMENT OF ADJUSTMENT PROBLEMS IN A PRISON SETTING

The consequences of nontreatment of adjustment problems in a prison setting can be severe. Emotional problems can lead to suicide attempts and conduct problems can threaten the safety of staff and other inmates or otherwise endanger the security of the institution. If left untreated, adjustment problems and Adjustment Disorders can persist indefinitely and develop into other Axis I disorders, potentially resulting in greater time (e.g., more treatment), expense (e.g., medications), and investment on the part of the staff and the institution than if the adjustment problems had been treated expediently at discovery. Finally, problems with adjustment to prison can make some inmates vulnerable to victimization by other inmates. Because the prison administration has a duty to maintain the safety of all in its employment and custody, the treatment of mental disorders is of utmost importance in this setting (Hafemeister, Hall, & Dvoskin, 2001).

Despite the prevalence of adjustment problems in prison, there are currently no specified empirically validated treatments for Adjustment Disorders. Rather, in practice, adjustment problems may be treated based on what is most effective for their particular symptom constellation, such as Cognitive Behavioral Therapy (CBT) for Adjustment Disorder with Depressed Mood, exposure for Adjustment Disorder with certain anxiety symptoms, or anger management for Adjustment Disorder with Disturbance of Conduct. That is, treatment based on the associated symptoms reflects what is most effective for that particular full syndrome. These particular treatments are described in detail elsewhere, and the reader is referred to other works for further elaboration (see Nathan & Gorman, 1998, for a summary of empirically validated treatments for common disorders).

In many cases, however, what lay behind the myriad of symptoms associated with poor adjustment to prison is difficulty with coping skills and problem solving in interpersonal relating—issues that CBASP is designed to address. The relationship between coping skills, problem solving, and prison adjustment was investigated in prior literature. For example, inmates with a greater inventory of coping skills self-reported less difficulty with adjustment than those who claimed fewer coping skills, highlighting the importance of teaching such skills to the latter group to promote positive adjustment (Negy, Woods, & Carlson, 1997). A similar pattern of results was found with regard to problem-solving skills in inmate samples (Pugh, 1993). In the absence of treatment, however, characteristic ways of coping and resulting adjustment difficulties in prison inmates were shown to persist over time (Negy, 1995).

These coping and problem-solving deficits, perhaps present prior to incarceration, may become exacerbated due to a reduction in a sense of personal control that is associated with confinement. It has already been established that the correctional environment by design places restrictions on the individuals residing therein and results in a reduction in the amount of control over many aspects of daily life. For some, this reduction in control and the inability to make decisions about the course of one's life may lead to the inaccurate perception that all control over one's life is lost. Prior research indicates that an extremely external locus of control orientation in the newly incarcerated is linked to increased depressive symptomatology over time (Reitzel & Harju, 2000) and poorer overall adjustment to prison, as measured by higher stress-related problems, more infractions, and less involvement in programming opportunities (cf. Pugh, 1993).

However, although the prison environment restricts personal choices for the incarcerated individual, it also affords some autonomy in decision making. For example, an offender can choose how to interact with staff and peers and handle the inevitable disputes with others. Those initially sent to close, or maximum, custody can advance to medium or minimum custody as a result of exemplary behavior while in close custody and thus achieve greater levels of freedom and independence. Application of the Coping Survey Questionnaire (CSQ), the structural backbone of CBASP, may be especially helpful in correctional environments because these environments enhance the perception of a lack of personal control, whereas the CSQ is designed to highlight the degree of personal control a patient has in achieving a particular Desired Outcome (DO).

The following is a case example of a session using CBASP within a prison setting to illustrate the process and its applicability to this population. The problem faced in this scenario is not an uncommon illustration of the nature of the situations that an inmate having adjustment difficulty in prison may face on a daily basis. It should be noted that in the following session, no modifications to the CSQ were necessary for implementation, as would probably be typical for use in this setting.

⌒ Case Example 1 ⌒

George is a 46-year-old, White man with a primary diagnosis of Adjustment Disorder with Depressed Mood. His methods of coping with his environment were leading to passive-type adjustment problems. The following excerpt is taken from a session in therapy using CBASP:

Therapist: Okay, George, I see you've brought in your homework for today. Why don't you go ahead and read out loud the situation you've chosen.

George: Okay, I was standing in line in the chow hall yesterday for lunch, and three guys from my block just cut in front of me in line. I didn't say anything to them at all. Then later I was eating and minding my own business when one of them just walked right up to my plate and took my dessert and walked away. I didn't say anything ... just finished my food.

Therapist: That's a good example of a situation that we can look at in here. You've described the facts of the situation in a few sentences or less and described it in such a way that I would see it if I were a

12. CORRECTIONAL SETTINGS 195

fly on the wall . . . just observing what actually happened. Tell me what you were thinking during the situation.

George: One was I thought I was such a wimp that I deserved to be picked on. I also thought that I was pretty stupid for getting myself into prison in the first place to have to deal with all this stuff. Then I thought that from now on I should just skip eating in the chow hall.

Therapist: Those sound like good thoughts to work with. Now behaviors . . . how did you act or what did you say in the situation?

George: Well, I just stood there while they got in front of me and I guess I looked away from them and tried not to make eye contact. Then I did the same when they took my food.

Therapist: Tell me your desired outcome.

George: I wanted to stand up for myself.

Therapist: Tell me what standing up for yourself would have looked like.

George: Well, I would have said something to them when they cut in line and when they took my food. Something that would have stopped them from doing it, I guess.

Therapist: Okay, so your desired outcome was to stand up for yourself and say something to the guys to stop them from taking advantage of you, right? What was the actual outcome?

George: I got taken advantage of, lost my dessert and ended up spending the rest of my day in my room feeling like crap.

Therapist: Did you achieve your desired outcome in this situation?

George: Uh . . . no.

Therapist: Okay. That's important for us to note. Now let's look at each thought and behavior and see whether each was helpful or hurtful in reaching your desired outcome of standing up for yourself. Let's turn our attention to your thoughts now. Take the first thought: You thought you were such a wimp that you deserved to be picked on. Was that helpful or hurtful in achieving your desired outcome of standing up for yourself?

George: Hurtful. It made me feel weak. It made me feel less like sticking up for myself.

Therapist: Okay. How about your second thought about being stupid for getting into prison in the first place? Did that help you or hurt you in achieving your desired outcome of standing up for yourself?

George: It was hurtful. I guess it just distracted me from the issue of being taken advantage of and made me feel weak and stupid.

(Session continues)

At this point the session continued with a review of the patient's thoughts and behaviors and their helpfulness in achieving the DO. Thoughts and behaviors would next be individually altered by the patient in a manner that would increase the likelihood of achieving the DO. For example, the thought "I'm a wimp and deserved to be picked on" could be changed to "I'm a human being and deserved to be treated fairly." Likewise, the thought "I'm stupid for getting into prison in the first place" could be changed to "I shouldn't have gotten into prison in the first place, but I'm here now and I have to deal with this situation."

An alternative to George's passive behavior of allowing peers to take advantage of him might be similar to the response an inmate exhibiting active-type adjustment problems would generate: starting a physical fight with the inmate who cut in front of him. The suggestion of such a behavioral alternative might arise in the process of George's CSQ. Though different than the passive inaction that he actually chose in this situation, this active response is also maladaptive and can be addressed in the context of the CSQ. Doing so would likely reveal the presence of dual DOs in this situation. In George's case, the dual DOs might be to stand up for himself and also to avoid getting a disciplinary infraction for misbehavior in the process. Therefore, whereas punching the inmate/s who cut in front of George might have been helpful in standing up for himself, such action would have been inconsistent (i.e., hurtful) with his DO of staying out of trouble.

When it becomes clear to the therapist that a patient has dual DOs in a situation, it is usually best (and more salient) to allow the patient to come to this recognition unassisted. Having George explore all possible results of his suggested action of punching the inmate might result in the recognition that getting an infraction and possibly segregation time would not be acceptable to him. When recognition of dual outcomes by the patient does not seem imminent, however, the therapist may need to lead the patient in this direction (e.g., "So what would staff members do if you hit the inmate? How will that segregation time affect your custody evaluation? Is it okay with you that you lose medium custody for another 6 months because of your response to this guy? Oh, so you're saying that you also have a DO of not getting in trouble over this incident?")

When a patient specifies dual DOs, each step of the CSQ should be reviewed with reference to each of these DOs, respectively (i.e., examine each cognition and behavior to see if it was helpful or hurtful in attaining each of the DOs). In a prison setting, dual outcomes are common because patients may wish to act in a way that achieves an immediate DO (e.g., getting back at a harassing peer or staff member, pressuring a peer for items of value, such as cigarettes) at the expense of a more distant and less salient DO (e.g., avoiding misbehavior to increase chances of custody promotions, earning privileges or early release).

In the process of reviewing the CSQ, it is ideal if the patient generates both the cognitive and behavioral alternatives. However, in some cases, patients may not be able to generate appropriate alternatives to achieve one or both of their DOs. For example, some patients may have habits of responding in aggressive or antisocial ways to others and may be resistant to acknowledging effective alternatives. Likewise, many inmates lack assertiveness skills and vacillate between passivity and aggressiveness as typical reactions to ·interpersonal problem situations. If this is the case, some time must be spent on assertiveness training and realistic options for the use of such responses in the prison environment. It is also appropriate for the therapist to help in the brainstorming process of alternative thoughts and behaviors, subsequently allowing the patient to evaluate whether the generated alternatives are helpful or hurtful in achieving the DO.

CBASP can be used to elucidate helpful and goal-oriented alternatives to current behavior for patients who typically respond to (or cope with) their environment in either passive or active ways. In fact, whatever the specifics of the situation, the CSQ helps to set the stage for change by linking thoughts, behaviors and outcomes in the Person × Environment interaction, by increasing coping and problem-solving skills in interpersonal relating.

TREATMENT OF ADJUSTMENT PROBLEMS
IN FORENSIC HOSPITAL SETTINGS

Similar to a prison setting, commitment to a forensic hospital places considerable limitations on an individual's liberty and freedom. To be committed to a forensic hospital, an individual must be adjudicated as Incompetent to Proceed or Not Guilty by Reason of Insanity. Patients in these settings are likely to have been charged with a variety of crimes in addition to experiencing a variety of symptoms of mental illness. In most cases, these patients are suffering from an acute thought or mood disorder, such as Schizophrenia, Schizoaffective Disorder, Bipolar Disorder, or Psychotic Disorder Not Otherwise Specified. Symptoms of these disorders may include auditory and visual hallucinations, delusions, paranoia, aggressive behavior, disorientation, and disorganized thought processes. When these patients enter the courtroom, these symptoms often prompt the judge to recommend psychological evaluations, resulting in an involuntary commitment to a forensic hospital for some. Once committed, these patients are likely to be treated with psychotropic medication to manage the mood disorder or psychotic symptoms.

Once these patients become stabilized on the appropriate medications, in many cases, symptoms of depression, anxiety, or personality disorders (e.g., Antisocial, Borderline, Dependent) remain. Similar to a prison environment, many patients in this setting are forced to live under a strict set of rules and regulations. In addition, they are separated from loved ones and are experiencing a variety of losses, such as loss of social support, liberty, security, material possessions, and acceptance by society. Many patients in forensic hospitals have been severely mentally ill for a significant portion of their lives. As a result, many have exhausted their social support and financial resources. Many are homeless, a circumstance that poses an additional difficulty in treating these individuals inasmuch as the hospital may provide the most stable and safe environment they have experienced in a long time. Therefore, treatment must focus on problem solving and skill building to help these patients transition into the community following restoration of competency or conditional release.

The strategies of CBASP are particularly relevant to treatment within an inpatient forensic hospital in that the patient must learn to effectively interact with other residents and staff members to be released from the hospital. CBASP is well suited for this purpose.

CASE EXAMPLE 2

This case example illustrates the application of the CSQ within an inpatient forensic hospital and demonstrates the applicability of CBASP to this population. This patient, Fred, was considered to have made a poor adjustment to the forensic setting, primarily due to

12. CORRECTIONAL SETTINGS

altercations resulting from difficulty getting along with peers and staff. Although this individual meets criteria for severe mental illness as well as ASPD, the situation described in this example is likely to generalize to many individuals in this setting. It is noteworthy that this individual completed seven CSQs prior to the one used in this example, which may account for his cooperation in the process and relative ease at generating alternative interpretations and behaviors. Therapists should keep in mind that the initial sessions are likely to be more difficult for both the patient and the clinician.

Fred is a 28-year-old, White man with a primary diagnosis of Major Depressive Disorder with psychotic features (e.g., hallucinations, delusions) and an Axis II diagnosis of ASPD. Primarily due to the latter diagnosis, Fred's coping and problem-solving style has led to active-type adjustment problems. At the time CBASP began, he had been in the hospital for 4 months. His depressive and psychotic symptoms had been stabilized via antidepressant and antipsychotic medication, but his personality disorder symptoms remained (e.g., deceitfulness, irresponsibility, irritability). These symptoms appeared to be resulting in significant problems with appropriate adjustment. At the onset of treatment, Fred struggled to maintain his behavior, thereby compromising his restoration of competency to stand trial. The following is an excerpt taken from his fifth session:

Therapist: Okay, Fred. Let's get started. I see that you brought your homework with you today. Why don't you go ahead and describe the situation to me. Remember, try to be specific and limit it to three or four sentences.

Fred: Okay, this morning a man said good morning to me, and I was not in the mood to speak to anyone. So, he said, out the side of his mouth, something like, "I said good morning, you ugly fuck!"

Therapist: Okay, so let me make sure I have this down. This morning, one of the other residents said good morning to you, but you didn't feel like saying good morning to him, so you didn't say anything at all. He responded by repeating himself and adding in some profanity.

Fred: Yeah, that's about right.

Therapist: Let's move on to Step 2. What were your thoughts and interpretations about this situation? What did you write down on your homework for Step 2?

Fred:	Do you want me to just list them to you?
Therapist:	Yeah, that would be fine.
Fred:	I'm not obligated to tell anyone good morning, I ought to kick his ass, he doesn't know who he's talking to, and, no, I might hurt him, I'm changing, I just need to let it go.
Therapist:	Okay, good. Those are four good thoughts that we can work with. Now, on to Step 3. What were your behaviors? What did you do in this situation?
Fred:	I didn't do anything.
Therapist:	Did you say anything to him?
Fred:	Nope.
Therapist:	Were you looking at him? What was your body language?
Fred:	I wasn't really looking at him. I just tensed up, in case he came at me.
Therapist:	Okay. So you tensed up your body in preparation for a possible fight?
Fred:	Yeah.
Therapist:	Am I missing anything?
Fred:	Nope. That's pretty much all that happened.
Therapist:	Let's move on to Steps 4 and 5. What was your desired outcome? What did you want to happen?
Fred:	I didn't want it to happen at all.
Therapist:	What do you mean? You didn't want what to happen at all?
Fred:	I didn't want him to mouth off to me the way he did.
Therapist:	So what actually happened?
Fred:	He walked away.
Therapist:	So, did you get what you wanted?
Fred:	Nope.
Therapist:	Alright, Fred, let's figure this out. First, let's look at your interpretations. The first one you told me was that you thought "I'm not obligated to tell anyone good morning." Do you think that thought helped you or hurt you in getting your desired outcome of avoiding this situation all together?
Fred:	I don't think it hurt.
Therapist:	Let's think about it. You didn't want him to mouth off to you. Do you think that particular thought helped you to get that outcome?
Fred:	No, I guess not.
Therapist:	I don't think so either. What do you think you could have thought instead that may have helped you get the outcome you wanted?
Fred:	I don't know. He should have just left me alone.

12. CORRECTIONAL SETTINGS 201

Therapist: But is there anything that you can think of that may have helped you avoid him mouthing off to you?

Fred: (*pause*) I guess I could have thought that he was just being friendly.

Therapist: Great! I agree, that may have helped avoid the situation all together. It certainly would have affected your original reaction to him. What about the thought "I ought to kick his ass." Did that one help you or hurt you?

Fred: It's the same thing. No, it didn't help. I should have just thought he was being nice and been nice in return.

Therapist: You don't sound convinced.

Fred: You just don't understand. You don't know these people. They just mess with me all the time.

Therapist: Fred, I know this is difficult, but we've talked about this before. Whose is the only behavior you can control?

Fred: Mine, I know. I should have just said good morning to him.

Therapist: Okay, what about the thought "No, I might hurt him, I'm changing, I should just let it go"? Did that one help you or hurt you in avoiding the confrontation?

Fred: That one sounds good to me.

Therapist: I agree. That was a good one. As we've seen, you probably could have avoided him mouthing off to you all together, but after he did, I think this was an excellent thought. And definitely a lot different from how you used to react to things.

Fred: Yeah, the old me would have just knocked him out as soon as the words left his mouth!

Therapist: What about your behaviors? You said that you didn't respond, and you tensed up. Did doing that help you to avoid the situation?

Fred: No, like I said, I should have just said good morning.

Therapist: You're getting good at this! Are there any other things you could have said or done?

Fred: I guess I could have just told him right off the bat that I was in a bad mood.

Therapist: Yeah, I agree. That might have helped. What could you have changed about your body language?

Fred: I shouldn't have tensed up, but I was just trying to protect myself.

Therapist: What do you think tensing up says to the other person?

Fred: That I'm ready to fight.

Therapist: Yeah, so it probably would have been helpful to maintain a relaxed posture. Do you agree?

Fred:	Whatever you say, Doc.
Therapist:	Very funny. Okay, it's about time to wrap up. So what did you learn from this situation?
Fred:	I don't know. I just don't think this will work with these guys. It all sounds fine in here with you, but you just don't know what it's like out there.
Therapist:	You're right. I don't know what it's like out there. But how about this, why don't you try it out? The next time one of these guys makes a comment to you, no matter what it is, think about the things we've worked on in here. Try to use the helpful thoughts and behaviors, and see how they react. Can you do that?
Fred:	I'll try, but I doubt it will work.
Therapist:	All I ask is that you try. I'll see you next time.
Fred:	All right. See you later.

Fred's case clearly illustrates the possible use of CBASP with individuals in an inpatient forensic setting. Indeed, CBASP and the CSQ were effective in helping Fred manage his behavior within the hospital and significantly decreased the number of altercations he had with other patients and staff members. Fred began to understand the connection between his interpretations and behaviors and the outcomes of daily encounters with patients and staff members.

OBSTACLES TO TREATMENT

There are a number of obstacles correctional psychologists encounter in providing treatment to incarcerated patients. Some of these are not unique to the use of CBASP but rather apply to the provision of all mental health treatment in these environments. In short, therapists in correctional settings have much to do, little time, and many patients to treat. In their national survey of correctional psychologists, Boothby and Clements (2000) found that approximately 30% of correctional psychologists' time was spent engaging in various administrative tasks, whereas therapeutic treatment comprised only 26% of the therapists' time. Compared with the amount of time they would ideally like to spend in these activities, therapists reported wishing less time could be devoted to the former and more time devoted to the latter (Boothby & Clements, 2000). A complicating factor is the low treatment provider to patient ratio in correctional settings. Boothby and Clements (2000) estimated that there are 750 inmates to every psychologist and 2,000 inmates to every PhD-level psychologist in prison and forensic settings. Additionally, in forensic settings, there is often a limited amount of time that the patient is committed to the hospital. In the case of those patients found incompetent to proceed, the goal of the psychology staff is to restore the individual to competency in the least amount of time possible to process the individual through the criminal justice system. This results in a high turnaround rate in forensic admission units, forcing psychologists to spend a significant amount of time on intake and competency evaluations rather than on treatment.

With limited time and a host of demands placed on them, correctional psychologists may have to make treatment decisions that leave those with comparatively less severe symptomatology or disorders, such as Adjustment Disorders, to their own resources, so they can make time to treat those with more severe symptomatology or disorders, such as Major Depression or Psychotic Disorders. Likewise, there may exist pressure from custodial staff to devote large amounts of time to counseling the more disruptive inmates, such as those with Borderline Personality Disorder, whereas treating those individuals with a minor depressive reaction to incarceration may be viewed as secondary. Alternatively, correctional psychologists in some settings may be forced to spend a good deal of time engaging in crisis management, with a resulting decrease in the time remaining for ongoing therapy. Their ever-increasing case loads may not allow the luxury of weekly individual sessions for multiple patients. Psychologists must work to strike a balance between the needs of the individuals in their care and the needs of the custodial staff, on which they rely for protection while working in correctional environments. Because correctional psychologists currently spend approximately twice as much time conducting individual treatment as they do conducting group treatment, the incorporation of more group treatment programs where applicable may be a necessary change to maximize their patient contact (Boothby & Clements, 2000).

Another challenge to correctional psychologists when implementing any new treatments involves obtaining approval from correctional administration and supervisory staff. Correctional environments are often based on a hierarchical, military-like structure, whereby those at the top make decisions for those below. In such established environments, some who may prefer the status quo may not view the introduction of a new treatment program very enthusiastically. To be fair, in most correctional settings, especially prisons, the primary administrative responsibility of those at the top levels of management is to maintain security, and rightfully so. Treatment needs of the inhabitants of the prison may be seen as secondary to this aim, at least in terms of priorities for decision making about the implementation of change. Correctional psychologists who encounter difficulties in establishing new treatment programs must face this challenge and be prepared to make an empirically supported case for such, as well as pay heed to the concerns of administrative staff regarding security issues and, perhaps most important, the cost-effectiveness of the proposed changes over the long term. Correctional settings, after all, legally have a dual mandate to both protect the public from offenders and also to provide mental health treatment to those in their keep who are in need of such (Wettstein, 1998).

Finally, the nature of correctional clientele may potentially be an obstacle to treatment. A correctional clinician is likely to come across a high degree of comorbidity, especially on Axis II, in such an environment. Comorbidity in general, and personality disorders in particular, may interfere with treatment in a number of ways. Correctional clinicians should be aware of this complicating factor and recognize that treatment may need to be altered accordingly (e.g., allowing lengthened treatment duration for some individuals). In addition, patients in correctional settings can be less than cooperative. This may be a result of Axis II symptomatology (e.g., problems with authority or manipulation), influence or fear of other inmates, or low levels of cognitive and intellectual functioning, which are all common in these settings. Therefore, correctional psychologists face the additional challenge of establishing a therapeutic relationship with these inmates and patients and earning their trust despite these barriers. Once a therapeutic relationship has been established, the CBASP approach is likely to be an effective tool for motivating these individuals and treating the variety of Axis I and II symptomatology that is likely to occur in these settings.

In conclusion, we believe it is reasonable to surmise, based on conceptual and applied grounds, that the tools of CBASP are ones particularly effective for use in the treatment of various disorders within correctional settings. The CSQ helps to elucidate the Person × Environment interaction and emphasize the personal control one has in achieving a reasonable DO in settings specifically designed to minimize perceptions of personal autonomy. In this chapter, the use of the CSQ was limited to the treatment of adjustment problems (e.g., Adjustment Disorders and related sequelae) in correctional settings, but we do not mean to suggest exclusivity of this diagnostic application. Indeed, CBASP and the CSQ are likely to be beneficial in the treatment of any number of disorders and may be particularly helpful in addressing interpersonal problems and conflicts that have their roots in problem solving, coping skills, and emotional regulation deficits.

Chapter **13**

The Cognitive Behavioral Analysis System of Psychotherapy: Future Directions*

> The major themes of each of the chapters in the book are summarized here. In addition, future directions for the Cognitive Behavioral Analysis System of Psychotherapy are proposed with regards both to research and to clinical practice.

This collection of practical guidelines and elucidatory case examples has made clear, we hope, the potential of the Cognitive Behavioral Analysis System of Psychotherapy (CBASP) approach. CBASP provides a simple, straightforward means by which clinicians can conceptualize and effectively treat some of the most complex, pernicious, even intractable psychological problems. In the following discussion, we show that although the chapters may describe quite disparate conditions, the clinical efforts reported herein cohere along several important common lines. These commonalities certainly account for the wide versatility and merit of CBASP, but they may also present a double-edged sword in its implementation in some situations. We offer some strategies for addressing these potential roadblocks. Finally, the flexibility afforded by CBASP permits our speculation about its adaptation to other psychological conditions and further allows us to elaborate on potentially fruitful avenues of research concerning its clinical use.

---

*The primary authors contributing to this chapter were Maureen Lyons Reardon, Kimberly A. Driscoll, Donald R. Kerr, Jr., and Thomas E. Joiner, Jr.

207

COMMON FEATURES

Although not explicitly stated in the chapters of this book, one of the more appealing aspects of CBASP repeatedly affirmed in this book is its emphasis on the formation of, and progress toward, goals. Such a focus arguably serves to motivate change in the targets of intervention and constitutes a refreshing alternative to traditional psychotherapy. Whereas many therapies often tend to assist patients to cope with or perhaps work through life's past and present struggles, CBASP encourages patients to work toward achieving what they actually desire in life. Obviating a belabored focus on the past, CBASP allows patients to begin therapy with an encouraging focus on their current Desired Outcomes (DOs). It is this optimistic spin on treatment that can make it quite desirable for those embittered by the failures of previous therapies. Indeed, a rather inspiring therapeutic atmosphere can be fostered by the therapist who praises patients for successfully attained outcomes.

In this way, CBASP serves to promote collaboration: The therapist and the patient work together to achieve therapeutic goals. As noted in several of the previous chapters, the relationship between therapist and patient may provide clinically useful material for in-session situational analysis, particularly for those patients whose interpersonal skills are considered inadequate or maladaptive. Inasmuch as psychological disorders are essentially defined by deviations from social norms, it is perhaps unsurprising that social situations have been afforded special importance in the proposed CBASP interventions. It is simply the relative emphasis placed on certain aspects of interpersonal functioning that vary with each patient's presenting problems. Whereas exposure to social interactions may be encouraged or even prescribed for certain conditions (e.g., Social Phobia, Schizotypal Personality Disorder—STPD), others may require social skills training (e.g., children with externalizing disorders, STPD) or perhaps work toward the development of more socially appropriate means of social communication (e.g., Borderline Personality Disorder, Anger Management, Couples Therapy). In other words, assisting patients to achieve their goals in the context of CBASP may necessitate the exposure to, knowledge of, and skills for following the conventions of social communication.

To some degree, CBASP is psychoeducational. As noted in each of the chapters, the process of Situational Analysis (SA) is presented to the patient at the outset of treatment in the structured form of the Coping Survey

Questionnaire (CSQ). As part of this instruction, the therapist first teaches the patient how to identify a realistically attainable goal and next encourages the patient to deduce what helps and what hurts with regard to that DO. In this sense, the identification of, and progress toward, goals may be considered a skill; one that can be learned, practiced, and developed through CBASP interventions. Step by step, patients may then learn to better navigate troubling interpersonal situations in an adaptive, appropriate manner. Moreover, because patients are granted the responsibility of identifying what helps and hurts with regard to their DO, successfully attained outcomes may be internally attributed. Repeated successes are bound to yield a sense of self-efficacy that supplants feelings of helplessness that often hinder progress in therapy. In this sense, CBASP promotes the patient's reliance on self, rather than on the therapist, as the agent of change, which may increase the likelihood that insights gained in session will be generalized outside of the therapy setting.

Thus far, we have shown that applications of CBASP to the psychological problems addressed in this book have several features in common. Yet how is it that such diverse problems, ranging from individual work with severe personality disorders to group work with parents of children with behavior problems to mood and anxiety disorders, are amenable to the present treatment with so much in common? One likely reason for the applicability of CBASP to such a wide range of psychological problems is that its cognitive and interpersonal foci, employing the simple CSQ, jibe well with empirically validated treatments (EVTs). Indeed, most treatments in the lists of those that are empirically validated or promising are Cognitive Behavioral or Interpersonal (e.g., Hollon & Beck, 1994; Nathan & Gorman, 1998) and readily lend themselves to the lean and flexible CBASP, which introduces little extra jargon or theory. In this sense, CBASP can provide practical guidance concerning the day-to-day implementation of EVTs, which is often lacking in many manualized protocols.

Thus, importantly, existing EVTs for many of the disorders presented in this text (Borderline Personality Disorder, Social Anxiety Disorder, Panic Disorder) need not be replaced by CBASP, but may be simply placed in its structured context (i.e., via the CSQ). Accordingly, we have advocated for the integration of the components or stylistic elements of existing therapies (e.g., Dialectical Behavioral Therapy, social skills training, relaxation, exposure) into CBASP. For example, the empirically validated use of anxiety ratings (SUDS) was incorporated into proposed adaptations of the CSQ for Social Anxiety Disorder. SUDS ratings may be used to select prescribed exposure and may further constitute a quantitative means by which attainment of a DO may be indexed (e.g., "I would like to ask her out on a date with only moderate anxiety," SUDS = 40).

POTENTIAL PITFALLS TO IMPLEMENTATION

Unfortunately, despite its strengths, including a tendency toward reduced reactance and defensiveness and increased collaboration, our CBASP applications can run onto rocky ground. As with any treatment approach, some clients do not respond constructively. Inherent in the process of encouraging patients to focus on their aspirations is the prerequisite that these goals exist. Yet for many the prospect of identifying or even expressing a DO can be daunting. Some persons may be unaccustomed to perceiving life situations in this manner or, for a variety of reasons, may be reluctant to assert themselves. Thus, in some instances, we had to make the initial therapeutic goal one of shaping behavior so that the patient could eventually participate in CBASP treatment.

Although simplicity is one of CBASP's more important virtues, that simplicity could actually turn off some patients. One professional said, "I can see that it might be useful to develop this skill, but my problems are much too complicated for that approach." Some such patients may respond positively to the therapist's plea to trust the therapist and try the approach. Others may be more resistant to the approach. One 60-year-old man with Narcissistic Personality Disorder and comorbid Dysthmic Disorder, for example, described the CSQ as "nickel-and-dime therapy" that was "beneath [him]." In this case, the therapist persisted, emphasizing the importance of homework completion, establishing the rapport necessary for his trust in the use of the therapist's interventions, while simultaneously gently challenging his impatience with therapy in the face of refusal to participate in recommended treatment. Despite his reluctance, the patient's Beck Depression Inventory scores decreased from 15 to 11 over the next several sessions. Thus, when faced with similar situations, we caution the therapist not to renounce the approach entirely but rather to apply these techniques more informally to interpersonal situations that will undoubtedly arise. There is at least some anecdotal support for the notion that the structure afforded by CBASP may be therapeutic in and of itself, especially for persons who may be ill adept to regulate their cognitions or emotions. The therapist would be best to remain mindful of the method,

13. FUTURE DIRECTIONS 211

using the steps outlined in the CSQ to guide the process of the therapy session.

It has been our experience that many patients engage in the process of therapy with the same interpersonal behaviors that necessitated their intervention in the first place. Tangents, emotional outbursts, and inconsistent homework and attendance can interrupt therapy. However, we assert that these behaviors can be effectively addressed by CBASP. In some ways, for example, CBASP naturally places the therapist in a kind of authoritative role: introducing the CSQ, teaching the method, and assigning similar homework week after week. Thus, patients who struggle with authority may find particular difficulty collaborating in such a setting. One such patient digressed, questioned, missed sessions, threatened termination, and chose superficial situations to analyze—all in a seemingly desperate attempt to undermine the CBASP. Using the method informally on in-session interactions enabled the patient to see how her behavior was undermining therapy just as it was undermining her performance throughout her life. Therapy prospered thereafter.

This apparent capacity to address therapy-interfering behaviors as targets of intervention speaks to one of the major assets of the CBASP approach, that is, the ease with which the approach can be adapted to address widely variable conditions and populations. Its wide versatility is clearly evident in Table 13.1, which highlights the key treatment guidelines proposed in the preceding chapters. Although some problems (e.g., Panic Disorder, Generalized Anxiety Disorder, correctional issues) may be effectively addressed with little to no alteration of the methods proposed by McCullough (2000), others may require special accommodation.

Fortunately, such modifications are facilitated by the immense flexibility of the CBASP approach. For example, some therapists have incorporated additional steps to the CSQ. As one example, because many persons with anger problems evince a particular difficulty identifying any nonangry feelings, Burns and White (chap. 11) advocate for adding an item to the CSQ to explicitly highlight the contribution of other emotions (e.g., sadness) to situations in which maladaptive interpersonal functioning is evident. Others supplement critically important ratings into the steps of the CSQ to better address specific targets of intervention. For example, SUDS ratings may be included as part of a specified DO for persons with Social Anxiety Disorder, whereas ratings of the relevance of a particular thought may help to address the tangential thought processes of persons with Schizotypal Personality Disorder in the context of CSQ (see chap. 2).

TABLE 13.1
Summary of Key Points of CBASP Chapters

Diagnosis	CBASP: Guidelines for SA	Modifications to CSQ Format
Part I: Personality Disorders		
Schizotypal	CBASP is directive, structured, and time limited. CBASP combines social skills training, reality testing, and interpersonal boundary reinforcement in the context of a refined CSQ.	Items are reordered with narrowly specified instructions; relevance of cognitions are rated (1–10). Analysis focuses on non-verbal social presentation, self-image and self-efficacy.
Borderline	CBASP incorporates stylistic elements of DBT, including social skills training and regular monitoring for suicidal ideation. Therapy-interfering behaviors are addressed as in-session CSQ.	No modification to structure of CSQ format is needed. Analysis focuses on thoughts of loss, mistrust, and guilt as well as self-image, and maladaptive interpersonal behaviors.
Passive-aggressive (negativistic)	Therapeutic relationship used to examine passive-aggressive tendencies addressed in CBASP. Failure to complete CSQ as possible passive-aggressive behavior is addressed.	No modification to structure of CSQ format is needed. Analysis focuses on the underlying negativistic motivation for behaviors.
NOS	CBASP is modified according to specific target maladaptive thoughts and behaviors.	Central focus is personalized and prioritized according to the individuals' maladaptive personality symptoms (thoughts and behaviors).
Part II: Anxiety Disorders		
Social Anxiety	Therapy integrates CBASP with exposure therapy. Situations analyzed are prescribed by the therapist as exposure assignments.	Performance and interpersonal situations are selected as exposure. CSQ incorporates ratings of subjective anxiety level. DO can be fixed to exposure with a desired target anxiety level.
Panic	Panic control treatment is used in combination with CBASP.	Emphasis is placed on the DO of avoided/endured panic. No modification to format of CSQ is necessary.
GAD	CBASP, with a problem-solving, goal-oriented purpose is used. The focus is on a specific worry.	Emphasis is placed on worry cognitions as avoidance behaviors. No modification to format of CSQ is necessary.

(Continued)

13. FUTURE DIRECTIONS

213

TABLE 13.1 *(Continued)*

Diagnosis	CBASP: Guidelines for SA	Modifications to CSQ Format
Part III: Parents, Children, and Couples		
Parents	Parent management training and cognitive problem-solving skills training is implemented within a group format.	Situations are chosen related to child behavior, and analyses emphasize social learning principles that underlie parent management training and cognitive underpinnings of problem-solving skills training.
Children	Didactic training regarding social skills and role plays within a group setting, including empathy instruction is used. Other group members and therapists provide feedback on behaviors and the steps of situational analysis.	CBASP uses simplified language for Situational Analysis, including additional items that evaluate the cause of the problem, empathy training, and anticipation and prevention of negative consequences.
Couples	CBASP integrates full assessment of primary problem area and openly provides a conceptualization of the problem to the couple. A 12-week commitment from both members is expected.	The couples' collective DO in a situation is examined. Individual members of the couple independently complete the CSQ for the same situation. The therapist examines discrepancies in DOs for a situation.
Part IV: Other Applications		
Anger management	Therapy addresses the physiological and emotional components of anger in a nonconfrontational manner. Relaxation techniques are incorporated. Role plays are used to evaluate nonverbal behaviors or to address minimization distortions.	Therapy includes an additional feeling step to explore the multiple components of anger. Differentiates between short-term (impulsive) and long-term DOs.
Correctional settings	The focus is on adaptive functioning in an institutional setting.	No modifications are necessary.

Additionally, for those patients who may be cognitively compromised as a function of their psychological symptoms (e.g., Schizotypal) or development (i.e., children), alteration of the content of the CSQ procedures may be considered. By revising the wording or breaking down some of the original CSQ items into several, more simplified steps, the specialized needs of these populations may be better met.

Importantly, CBASP does not require that complex theoretical constructs be used to develop the conceptual framework needed to modify the approach for various conditions. Once familiar with the basic tenets of CBASP outlined previously and in the introductory chapter of this book, it becomes quite easy to imagine how this method might be applied to any number of problems. Indeed, it could be argued that a limitation of this text is its failure to provide an exhaustive presentation of the full range of psychological problems that would probably benefit from CBASP. This is due, at least in part, to constraints on the availability of experiences with its application as a function of our clinic population. However, given its apparent versatility, it seems reasonable to expect that CBASP may be used to address several other targets of intervention, an issue we shall consider next.

CLINICAL IMPLICATIONS FOR THE TREATMENT OF OTHER DISORDERS

In this section, we offer some suggestions for how CBASP might be modified to address some other psychological problems not presented in the preceding chapters. These speculations should not be considered as all-inclusive guidelines for CBASP application to these disorders or problems but rather as skeletal frameworks that require some fleshing out by the innovative therapist with due consideration of available science and the patient's individual needs.

We have already shown that CBASP may be an effective tool for improving emotional regulation, including states of depression (McCullough, 2000). As psychoactive substance use is often purposed as a means, albeit a maladaptive and temporary one, to manage emotional states (e.g., decrease depression, cope with anxiety, tune out), it seems reasonable to expect that CBASP may be useful in the treatment of Substance Use Disorders (SUD) as well. Indeed, poor emotional regulation in the context of a high-risk situation can often lead to relapse following a period of abstinence (Monti & Rohsenow, 1999). Thus, by improving management of emotions in a situation-specific manner, CBASP may effectively reduce the likelihood of relapse in persons recovering from SUD. The social skills training aspects of CBASP may also effectively decrease the stress associated with ineffective or maladaptive interpersonal functioning, which can also lead to relapse in this population (Monti & Rohsenow, 1999). In many ways, CBASP

13. FUTURE DIRECTIONS   215

is similar to existing SUD treatments that target areas of functioning that are indirectly related to substance use (e.g., Longabaugh & Morgenstern, 1999) or that place persons at risk for relapse (e.g., Fuller & Hiller-Sturmöfel, 1999; Irwin, Bowers, Dunn, & Wang, 1999).

Moreover, the relative emphasis on substance-related consequences in the diagnostic criteria for SUD lends itself well to CBASP intervention, which affords a similar prominence to outcomes. That is, SUDs are defined not by the quantity or frequency of use, but rather by its associated impact on the legal, interpersonal, occupational, and health-related domains of functioning (American Psychiatric Association, 1994). Furthermore, problem-solving approaches to SUD may be preferable to more traditional therapies that do not involve skill acquisition or other behavioral tactics, in that the former (e.g., relapse prevention) tend to generalize and gain effectiveness with time, whereas the latter (e.g., aversive counterconditioning) may lose effectiveness (Miller, 1978; Walters, 2000). To the degree that CBASP facilitates the patient's arrival at the cognitive and behavioral means to a certain desirable end (e.g., cessation or curtailment of use, harm avoidance), the method can be said to involve problem-solving tactics.

Indeed, existing SUD treatments, which incorporate cognitive and behavioral strategies (Hollon & Beck, 1994), are easily integrated into CBASP. For example, Harm Reduction Therapy (Marlatt, 1998) calls for the examination of the positive and negative consequences of substance use in an effort to decrease or alter use so as to decrease the likelihood of adverse consequences. In the context of CBASP via the CSQ, these positive or negative consequences may simply be considered Actual Outcomes (AO) that are either consistent or inconsistent with the DO to avoid psychosocial disruption due to substance use, respectively. Thus, through CBASP techniques, connections between substance use (a behavior) and its interference with positive psychosocial outcomes may be elucidated. Such connections may be critical for making adaptive decisions regarding both the initiation of substance use and the curtailment of use once an episode of consumption has commenced (Breiner, Stritzke, & Lang, 1999).

CBASP also dovetails nicely with Motivational Interviewing/Enhancement approaches to SUD (Miller & Rollnick, 1991), which hold as basic tenets the avoidance of argumentation (confrontation) and promotion of change. Borrowing from Prochaska, DiClemente, and Norcross's (1997) stages of change model, motivational therapies aim to meet the patients where they are in their recovery and gently move them toward elimination of their problematic substance use by helping them appreciate the discrepancy between where their life is (i.e., the AO) and where they would like it to be (i.e., the DO). Thus, depending on the patient's stage of change, CBASP may involve several possible DOs, for which failed or successful attainment may result in either addiction or a step toward recovery, respectively.

At the precontemplation stage, for example, patients often do not see the contribution of their substance use to their psychosocial disruption and are therefore not considering change in their substance use patterns (Miller & Rollnick, 1991). At this very early stage of recovery, the CSQ may be used to reveal that, for example, the behavior of substance use hurts the patient in achieving the DO of having a nice anniversary dinner with his wife. Successive examination of situations may ultimately reveal, in a nonconfrontational way, that substance use is a recurrent behavioral factor that contributes to repeated unsuccessful outcomes. This revelation may then move persons toward the contemplation stage of change, where cessation or reduction of use may be considered, albeit ambivalently. Alternate DOs may be involved at later stages of change (e.g., action and maintenance), where avoidance of relapse becomes key. At these stages, CBASP can help to reveal the cognitive (e.g., feelings of worthlessness, helplessness) and behavioral (e.g., going to a bar, fighting with spouse) factors that contribute to relapse—that is, the failure to achieve the DO of sobriety. Thus, in many ways, CBASP may serve as an effective relapse prevention approach.

Borrowing from these possible applications to SUD treatment, appetitive behaviors, such as sexual addiction, compulsive gambling, and overeating, may also be similarly addressed by CBASP interventions.

Moreover, given our experience that CBASP can enhance many cognitive behavioral and interpersonal therapies, it seems reasonable to expect that this treatment may also be applicable to those conditions for which these treatments have been empirically validated. For example, despite a history of intractability, eating disorders, particularly bulimia, have been shown to benefit from these interventions (e.g., Fairburn, Jones, Hope, & O'Connor, 1993; Wilson & Fairburn, 1998). In fact, we did have a truncated experience using CBASP with a person diagnosed with anorexia, who presented for treatment in the midst of a suicide crisis. This young college graduate had been in various treatments involving multiple hospitalizations, with seemingly little impact on her maladaptive behaviors. Because she reportedly had not been responsive to cognitive behavioral treatment, we opted for an Interpersonal Psychotherapy approach, en-

13. FUTURE DIRECTIONS

hanced by CBASP. The patient, who was initially very anxious and unfocused, found that prospective CSQs led to unprecedented successful encounters with her parents. This motivated her to work harder in therapy, which, in turn, resulted in other clinically important gains, including increased self-confidence.

Perhaps unfortunately for the patient as well as our experience base, she applied her newly gained assertiveness to find a job elsewhere and moved. Still, we came away from that experience optimistic about the usefulness of CBASP for eating disorders, provided its consistent focus on interpersonal functioning. In connection with more traditional cognitive behavioral approaches to eating disorders, CBASP may also be used to reveal how the cognitive distortions (e.g., self-hatred, overestimation of one's size, inaccurate size comparison with others) can contribute to self-deprivation, binge eating, or maladaptive compensatory strategies (purging, excessive exercise), which, in turn, interfere with adaptive functioning (DO).

Just as regulation of emotions is tantamount to the treatment of many psychological disorders (e.g., substance abuse, depression), learning to regulate life-management skills is critical to the treatment of neurobehavioral disorders, such as Attention-Deficit/Hyperactivity Disorder (ADHD). Due to the nature of the ADHD symptoms, patients with the disorder are often void of structure and direction. This, in turn, may result in problematic interpersonal relationships and difficulties fulfilling responsibilities at work and at school. Nadeau (1995) recommends several areas that need to be improved when managing the symptoms of ADHD. These include attention, memory, problem solving, time management, organization of the environment, and stress reduction. In this connection, CBASP provides a structured and focused approach for managing just the sorts of challenges with which patients with ADHD are presented.

Likewise, given that persons with specific learning disorders often experience some of the same life-management problems as patients with ADHD, they could also benefit from CBASP. For example, time management and the use of compensatory strategies (i.e., capitalizing on strengths in specific learning modalities, visual vs. auditory) are often problematic for patients with specific learning disorders. The CBASP approach allows the patient to analyze specific situations in terms of DOs and AOs with the ultimate goal being the modification of maladaptive behaviors. A patient who has been reprimanded at work or who has failed a test can easily analyze the situation in terms of the behaviors that contributed to the negative outcome. Formulating alternative behaviors (e.g., applying study skills, not procrastinating) highlights for the patient those behaviors that need to be changed to attain the DO (e.g., not being reprimanded or passing a test). In addition, the improvement of memory skills can easily be demonstrated by analyzing situations in which forgetfulness is particularly problematic. Developing compensatory strategies for improving memory (e.g., making lists, using a calendar for scheduling) are approaches that will likely reveal themselves as helpful through the use of SA.

As a method for promoting adaptive, compensatory strategies for accommodating restrictions imposed by psychological conditions such as learning disorders, it seems CBASP may have something to offer in connection with a wide variety of psychological problems that fall within the realm of health psychology. These include preoperative preparation, treatment adherence (e.g., medicine or physical therapy), psychological adjustment to a medical condition, chronic pain control, and problems related to aging. In the case of treatment adherence, a coexisting psychological condition (personality disorders, anxiety, etc.) can interfere with treatments, such as insulin injection. We showed that CBASP works for many of these disorders and thus may be applicable here. Accidents and ailments can give rise to such adjustment reactions as depression, anxiety, and behavior problems that can certainly be addressed by CBASP. To some degree, the recommendations offered in connection with adjustment to incarceration (chap. 12) may also be applicable to learning to adapt to the confines and restrictions imposed by a cooccurring medical condition. Additionally, CBASP may well be instrumental in behavioral activation related to pain (e.g., examining cognitions that interfere with attaining the goal of physical exercise). Persons with closed head injuries may also profit from using SA to help interpret interactions and events in their new and at times unfamiliar world.

Aging brings its own situations and interpersonal problems. Successful adaptation to age-related changes probably involves cognitive (e.g., positive attributions, sense of self-efficacy, future orientation) and behavioral adjustments (e.g., coping, social/community involvement) that should be tractable to CBASP intervention. It should be noted that with aging comes memory problems and other cognitive difficulties that may interfere with the analytic process. Elaboration on the worksheet of the CSQ, for example, may reduce demands on memory that might otherwise hinder more traditional, less-structured psychotherapies.

At first glance, it may seem that CBASP is less amenable to some psychological conditions, particularly those in which psychotropic medications are clearly the preferred mode of treatment (e.g., Schizophrenia, Bipolar

Disorder). However, this should not preclude the use of CBASP as a potential adjunct intervention for these disorders. Indeed, there exist pervasive problems with medication compliance among persons with these conditions that certainly can lead to undesirable outcomes, such as decompensation and rehospitalization.

For some, the use of medications may be perceived as a crutch. Others may simply find the medication side effects unbearable or perhaps a hindrance to the enhanced productivity afforded by episodes of hypomania. With regard to these issues, CBASP can be used to show that such thoughts lead directly to noncompliance with treatment regimens, which, in turn, results in unintended adverse consequences. For those psychological conditions characterized by symptomatic cognitive deficits (e.g., Schizophrenia), failure to comply with medications (behavior) may reflect something other than a calculated choice process. Fortunately, this can also be handled in the context of CBASP. The process of CBASP shows, in a very concrete and uncomplicated way, that medication noncompliance consistently hurts in the achievement of DOs of, say, independent community living (rehospitalization). Moreover, once medication compliance is secure, CBASP may still prove useful for many schizophrenics, who present with social skills deficits and oddities of behavior that compromise their ability to function effectively in community settings. For this purpose, many of the accommodations recommended for the treatment of Schizotypal Personality Disorder, as outlined in chapter 2, may prove useful.

A possible consequence of the wide impact of CBASP is the blurring of the lines between psychiatric diagnoses. With personality disorders in particular, it may be that the inability to interact effectively in interpersonal situations is the essential deficit—an inability, of course, which is the target of CBASP interventions. This may suggest use of CBASP with persons presenting narcissistic or even antisocial personality disorders, conditions that have a history of intractability. Essentially, CBASP evaluates what prevents patients from getting what they want in life—an aim that effectively cuts across any delineation as a function of diagnostic category.

In this sense, CBASP may facilitate interventions with persons suffering from two or more co-occurring psychological conditions. Although many practitioners may hold that integrated, as opposed to parallel (treating each disorder separately but concurrently) or serial (treating one disorder, then the next), approach is optimal—particularly for disorders comorbid with SUD (e.g., Johnson, 1992; Miller, Leukefeld, & Jefferson, 1996)—these notions have not apparently benefited from much growth of research in this area (Room, 1998). Thus, there presently exists little consensus concerning the effective treatment of comorbid disorders, and this remains a contentious area. Yet we showed that a multitude of psychological conditions may be effectively addressed with CBASP. CBASP encompasses a broad-sweeping attack on key hindrances to adaptive functioning (e.g., inadequate goal orientation, poor interpersonal functioning) and thus may be better able to accommodate comorbid conditions. The therapist may select from CBASP guidelines for the various disorders presented in this text (see Table 13.1) those that best accommodate the patient's unique presenting issues, regardless of what disorder these problems may have been generated from. Chapter 6, for example, provides a good example of how comorbid depressive symptoms were effectively addressed in a patient with primary Social Anxiety Disorder.

Finally, it seems likely that given its versatility and flexibility, the CBASP approach may be well applied in the self-help domain, potentially reaching patients who are reluctant to pursue formal therapy. The approach is so simple and straightforward that it seems reasonable to expect that many patients could benefit from its presentation in a self-help format. We can envision a text describing the approach that offers examples of various situations with desirable or undesirable outcomes, accompanied by an activity workbook that guides the reader through CSQ assignments addressing a variety of life situations (e.g., job interviews, arguments with family or children, financial problems).

In many ways, CBASP is a practical problem-solving approach to life that can be broadly applied. Although the wider application of CBASP was generated in an outpatient university-based psychology clinic, the chapters in this text clearly illustrate the applicability of this approach to a variety of settings and with a variety of conditions. We hope to promote use of CBASP (in conjunction with other empirically validated techniques) with disorders not necessarily outlined in this book and strongly encourage research designed to demonstrate its efficacy across the full spectrum of psychological disorders.

RESEARCH IMPLICATIONS

Although CBASP has been demonstrated an effective treatment of chronic depression (McCullough, 2000), it is openly acknowledged that evidence in support for the use of this approach for the range of conditions dis-

13. FUTURE DIRECTIONS

cussed in this text falls short of what would be desirable. Some of the proposed modifications to CBASP are speculations, based in part on extrapolations from our clinical experiences. Nonetheless, on the basis of actual cases in which CBASP was successfully implemented, we presented some compelling anecdotal evidence for its potential use for a variety of psychological problems and disorders. Although our findings await more systematic empirical validation, the hypotheses generated in the pages of this text should provide a solid basis for future efforts along these lines. In partial fulfillment of the criteria needed to establish CBASP as an EVT for these disorders, the series of cases presented here were based on a manualized protocol and included clearly defined target populations. We implore the reader to follow our lead and test our predictions empirically.

On a somewhat less-formal level, clinicians could simply test the approach with their own patients and evaluate its effectiveness for themselves. Ideally, these clinicians would then report the results to the practicing community as we have here. Such case study reports can be quite persuasive, particularly if several of them are published.

On a smaller scale, single subject study designs may be easily introduced into clinical practice (e.g., a simple interrupted time series, A-B). For example, a clinician who may appropriately use Dialectical Behavioral Therapy in her treatment of a patient suffering from Borderline Personality Disorder may, after a period of objective baseline assessment (A) on key targets of intervention (e.g., suicidal gestures, anger outbursts), introduce the CBASP method (B) as outlined in chapter 3. Clearly, the effects of CBASP are not instantaneous, and there is an expected time lag in its effectiveness (e.g., due to teaching and understanding of CSQ). Thus, the objective indices of target behaviors should be plotted graphically during baseline period, at expected time lag of say four sessions once CBASP is introduced, and for a period of several months of therapy thereafter. With these plotted data points, the clinician could empirically evaluate whether there was any change in the slope of the plot of target behaviors during the period following treatment, as compared to baseline. If a few more patients were available for evaluation, slopes could be compared among patients who were introduced to CBASP at point B to patients who continued to receive Dialectical Behavioral Therapy (DBT) treatment as usual. Alternately, the points at which CBASP was incorporated could be counterbalanced across patients. Another smaller scale design might involve the comparison of several patients who receive CBASP alone to those receiving DBT or CBASP-enhanced DBT.

Analyses such as these have the potential to show, in a systematic way, that changes in the key targets of intervention are indeed attributable to CBASP. Preferably, these smaller-scale studies would also include longer term, posttreatment follow-up assessment on key targets of intervention (e.g., at 6 months and 12 months). Objective analyses such as these would lend certain credibility to the anecdotal evidence presented in this text, and future efforts along these lines are forthcoming from our clinic.

Of course, larger scale group-design studies are better suited to address the therapeutic efficacy of CBASP for the various problems and disorders presented in this book. We can envision a series of pre-post, randomized control clinical trials, wherein global functioning or perhaps severity of target symptoms (e.g., anger outbursts) are assessed in well-defined clinical groups (e.g., persons with Panic Disorder) at the start of treatment, at its conclusion, and at prespecified follow-up intervals. Outcome indices (pre-post change) could then be compared across patients randomly assigned to treatment as usual or to CBASP, as proposed in this book. Assuming adherence to therapy protocols is adequately ensured, demonstrating that CBASP is superior to treatment as usual would lend support to its establishment as an empirically validated treatment for the target conditions. Other studies could compare groups of patients assigned to EVT or EVT and CBASP to evaluate the validity of our contention that integrating established EVTs into CBASP's more structured context may have clinical use for some conditions.

Investigations such as these have the potential to delineate possible boundaries for CBASP's efficacy, perhaps revealing that the methods of CBASP are effective in the alleviation of certain symptoms (e.g., interpersonal skills) or specific disorders, but not for others. This would help to establish important inclusion and exclusion criteria for the selection of patients who may be most likely to benefit from CBASP. Examination of the impact of CBASP on symptoms (e.g., substance abuse) other than those that constitute the focus of clinical attention (anxiety) may also help to answer whether the presence of comorbid conditions requires specific independent treatment—an issue of certain interest to the treatment community.

Once the efficacy of CBASP is established, process research could be pursued. For example, it might be interesting to determine how many CSQs are needed until successful outcomes are achieved. Does this depend on diagnosis, patient characteristics, or the quality of the therapeutic relationship? How many successful CSQs are needed before therapeutic efficacy is attained? How important are in-session CSQ evaluations, compared with therapies involving CSQs completed for homework? Other key questions involve the steps outlined in the CSQ as it relates to outcome. It may be important to evaluate whether the behavioral or cognitive changes have more impact on therapeutic outcome and whether or not this varies as a function of condition. This might suggest that certain disorders benefit from a greater therapeutic emphasis on behaviors than cognitions (e.g., as proposed for Schizotypal Personality Disorder in chap. 2), or vice versa.

Asking which features of the existing treatments into which we have integrated CBASP are needed for efficacy also may lead to some interesting studies. It is also important to determine whether or not the CBASP modifications proposed for certain disorders (i.e., added steps, ratings, and modified wording) are critical to treatment efficacy. It could be that the process of analyzing situations alone carries much of the variance in many of the applications that we have presented, a finding that could lead to even simpler treatments.

In this chapter, we summarized the ways in which we have applied the CBASP techniques to a number of problems other than depression. We demonstrated that our various approaches share several common features, including goal orientation, the promotion of collaboration, a focus on interpersonal functioning, and integration into existing treatments. The summary of treatment guidelines and CSQ modifications in Table 13.1 is a useful source for quick reference to the key material presented in this book.

We have also proposed that CBASP may be effective in treating several other problems and disorders. We feel there is now a solid basis for hypothesis generation relevant to empirical study, and, accordingly, we have offered some ideas for potentially fruitful avenues of empirical investigation.

References

Alberti, R. E., & Emmons, M. L. (1995). *Your perfect right: A guide to asssertive living* (25th ed.). Atascadero, CA: Impact Publishers.

American Psychiatric Association. (1980). *Diagnostic and statistical manual of mental disorders* (3rd ed.). Washington, DC: Author.

American Psychiatric Association. (1994). *Diagnostic and statistical manual of mental disorders* (4th ed.). Washington, DC: Author.

Asher, S. R. (1990). Recent advances in the study of peer rejection. In S. R. Asher & J. D. Coie (Eds.), *Peer rejection in childhood*. Cambridge, UK: Cambridge University Press.

Ballenger, J. C. (1999). Current treatments of the anxiety disorders in adults. *Biological Psychiatry, 46*, 1579–1594.

Barber, J., & Munez, L. (1996). The role of avoidance and obsessiveness in matching patients to cognitive and interpersonal psychotherapy: Empirical findings from the Treatment for Depression Collaborative Research Program. *Journal of Consulting and Clinical Psychology, 64*, 951–958.

Barkley, R. A. (1997). *Defiant children: A clinician's manual for assessment and parent training* (2nd ed.). New York: Guilford.

Barlow, D. H., & Craske, M. G. (1994). *Mastery of your anxiety and panic* (2nd ed.). Albany, NY: Graywind Publications.

Barlow, D. H., Esler, J. L., & Vitali, A. E. (1998). Psychosocial treatments for panic disorders, phobias, and generalized anxiety disorder. In P. E. Nathan & J. M. Gorman (Eds.), *A guide to treatments that work* (pp. 288–318). New York: Oxford University Press.

Barlow, D. H., Raffa, S. D., & Cohen, E. M. (2002). Psychosocial treatments for panic disorders, anxiety disorders, and generalized anxiety disorder. In P. E. Nathan & J. M. Gorman (Eds.), *A guide to treatments that work* (2nd ed., pp. 301–328). New York: Oxford University Press.

Baucom, D. H., Shoham, V., Mueser, K. T., Daiuto, A. D., & Stickle, T. R. (1998). Empirically supported couple and family interventions for marital distress and adult mental health problems. *Journal of Consulting and Clinical Psychology, 66*, 53–88.

Beck, A. T., & Freeman, A. (1990). *Cognitive behavioral therapy for personality disorders*. New York: Guilford.

Beck, A. T., & Rector, N. A. (2000). Cognitive therapy of schizophrenia: A new therapy for the new millennium. *American Journal of Psychotherapy, 54*(3), 291–300.

Beck, A. T., Rush, A. J., Shaw, B. F., & Emery, G. (1987). *Cognitive therapy of depression*. New York: Guilford.

Bellack, A., & Hersen, M. (1985). *Dictionary of behavior therapy techniques.* New York: Pergamon.

Benjamin, L. S. (1993). *Interpersonal diagnosis and treatment of personality disorders.* New York: Guilford.

Beutler, L., Mohr, D., Grawe, K., & Engel, D. (1991). Looking for differential treatment effects: Cross-cultural predictors of differential psychotherapy efficacy. *Journal of Psychotherapy Integration, 1,* 121–141.

Bloomquist, M. L. (1996). *Skills training for children with behavior disorders: A parent and therapist guidebook.* New York: Guilford.

Boothby, J., & Clements, C. (2000). A national survey of correctional psychologists. *Criminal Justice and Behavior, 27,* 716–732.

Borkovec, T. D., & Costello, E. (1993). Efficacy of applied relaxation and cognitive-behavioral therapy in the treatment of generalized anxiety disorder. *Journal of Consulting and Clinical Psychology, 61,* 611–619.

Breiner, M. J., Stritzke, W. G. K., & Lang, A. R. (1999). Approaching avoidance: A step essential to the understanding of craving. *Alcohol Health and Research World, 23,* 197–206.

Brestan, E. V., & Eyberg, S. M. (1998). Effective psychosocial treatment of conduct-disordered children and adolescents: 29 years, 82 studies, 5,275 children. *Journal of Clinical Child Psychology, 27,* 180–189.

Brosnan, R., & Carr, A. (2000). Adolescent conduct problems. In A. Carr (Ed.), *What works with children and adolescents: A critical review of psychological interventions with children, adolescents and their families* (pp. 131–154). London: Routledge.

Brown, E., Heimberg, R., & Juster, H. (1995). Social phobia subtype and avoidant personality disorder: Effect on severity of social phobia, impairment, and outcome of cognitive behavioral treatment. *Behavior Therapy, 26,* 467–486.

Brown, T. A., O'Leary, T. A., & Barlow, D. H. (1993). Cognitive-behavioral treatment of generalized anxiety disorder. In D. H. Barlow (Ed.), *Clinical handbook of psychological disorders* (2nd ed.). New York: Guilford Press.

Butler, G., Fennell, M., Robson, P., & Gelder, M. (1991). Comparison of behavior therapy and cognitive-behavior therapy in the treatment of generalized anxiety disorder. *Journal of Consulting and Clinical Psychology, 59,* 167–175.

Chambless, D. L., & Ollendick, T. H. (2000). Empirically supported psychological interventions: Controversies and evidence. *Annual Review of Psychology, 52,* 685–716.

Craske, M. G., & Barlow, D. H. (1992). Panic disorder and agoraphobia. In D. H. Barlow (Ed.), *Clinical handbook of psychological disorders* (2nd ed., pp. 1–47). New York: Guilford.

Crits-Christoph, P. (1998). Psychosocial treatments for personality disorders. In P. E. Nathan & J. M. Gorman (Eds.), *A guide to treatments that work* (pp. 3–25). New York: Oxford University Press.

Crits-Christoph, P., & Barber, J. (2002). Psychological treatments for personality disorders. In P. E. Nathan & J. M. Gorman (Eds.), *A guide to treatments that work* (2nd edition; pp. 611–623). New York: Oxford University Press.

Deffenbacher, J. L. (1999). Cognitive-behavioral conceptualization and treatment of anger. *Journal of Clinical Psychology, 55,* 295–309.

REFERENCES

227

Deffenbacher, J. L., Dahlen, E. R., Lynch, R. S., Morris, C. D., & Gowensmith, W. N. (2000). An application of Beck's cognitive therapy to general anger reduction. *Cognitive Therapy and Research, 24,* 689–697.

Ellis, A. (2001.) *Overcoming destructive beliefs, feelings, and behaviors: New directions for rational emotive behavior therapy.* Amherst, NY: Prometheus Books.

Estrada, A. U., & Pinsof, W. M. (1995). The effectiveness of family therapies for selected behavioral disorders of childhood. *Journal of Marital and Family Therapy, 21,* 403–440.

Fairburn, C. G., Jones, R., Hope, R. A., O'Connor, M. (1993). Psychotherapy and bulimia nervosa: Longer-term effects of interpersonal psychotherapy, behavior therapy, and cognitive behavior therapy. *Archives of General Psychiatry, 50,* 419–428.

Freeman, A., Pretzer, J., Fleming, B., & Simon, K. M. (1990). *Clinical applications of cognitive therapy.* New York: Plenum Press.

Fuller, R. K., & Hiller-Sturmöfel, S. (1999). Alcoholism treatment in the United States. *Alcohol Research and Health, 23,* 69–77.

Gabbard, G. O. (2000). *Psychodynamic Psychiatry* (3rd ed.). Washington, DC: American Psychiatric Press.

Gacono, C. B., Nieberding, R. J., Owen, A., Rubel, J., & Bodholdt, R. (2001) Treating conduct disorder, antisocial personality disorder, and psychopathic personalities. In J. B. Ashford, B. D. Sales, & W. H. Reid (Eds.), *Treating adult and juvenile offenders with special needs* (pp. 99–129). Washington, DC: American Psychological Association.

Gerzina, M. A., & Drummond, P. D. (2000). A multimodal cognitive-behavioural approach to anger reduction in an occupational sample. *Journal of Occupational and Organizational Psychology, 73,* 181–194.

Goldberg, S. C., Schultz, S. C., Schultz, P. M., Resnick, R. J., Hamer, R. M., & Friedel, R. O. (1986). Borderline and schitzotypal personality disorders treated with low-dose thiothixine vs. placebo. *Archives of General Psychiatry, 43,* 680–686.

Green, A. (1977). The borderline concept: A conceptual framework for the understanding of borderline patients: Suggested hypotheses. In P. Hartocollis (Ed.), *Borderline personality disorders: The concept, the syndrome, the patient* (pp. 15–44). New York: International Universities Press.

Greenberg, L. M., & Johnson, S. M. (1988). *Emotionally focused couples therapy.* New York: Guilford.

Haddock, G., Tarrier, N., Spaulding, W., Yusupoff, L., Kinney, C., & McCarthy, E. (1998). Individual cognitive-behavior therapy in the treatment of hallucinations and delusions: A review. *Clinical Psychology Review, 18,* 821–838.

Hafemeister, T. L., Hall, S. R., & Dvoskin, J. A. (2001). Administrative concerns associated with the treatment of offenders with mental illness. In J. B. Ashford, B. D. Sales, & W. H. Reid (Eds.), *Treating adult and juvenile offenders with special needs* (pp. 419–444). Washington, DC: American Psychological Association.

Hollon, S. D., & Beck, A. T. (1994). Cognitive and cognitive-behavioral therapies. In A. E. Bergin & S. L. Garfield (Eds.), *Handbook of psychotherapy and behavior change* (4th ed., pp. 428–466). New York: Wiley.

Hope, D. A., & Heimberg, R. G. (1993). SAD and social anxiety. In D. H. Barlow (Ed.), *Clinical handbook of psychological disorders: A step-by-step treatment manual* (2nd ed., pp. 99–136). New York: Guilford.

Hymowitz, P., Frances, A. J., Jacobsberg, L. B., Sickles, M., & Hoyt, R. (1986). Neuroleptic treatment of schizotypal personality disorders. *Comprehensive Psychiatry, 27,* 267–271.

Irwin, J. E., Bowers, C. A., Dunn, M. E., & Wang, M. C. (1999). Efficacy of relapse prevention: A meta-analytic review. *Journal of Consulting and Clinical Psychology, 67,* 563–570.

Johnson, R. A. (1992). Adapting the chronic disease model in the treatment of dually diagnosed patients. *Journal of Substance Abuse Treatment, 9,* 63–70.

Johnson, S., & Lebow, J. (2000). The "coming of age" of couple therapy: A decade review. *Journal of Marital and Family Therapy, 26,* 23–38.

Joiner, T., & Rudd, M. D. (2002). The incremental validity of passive-aggressive personality symptoms rivals or exceeds that of other personality symptoms in suicidal outpatients. *Journal of Personality Assessment, 79,* 161–170.

Joiner, T. E., Walker, R. L., Rudd, M. D., & Jobes, D. A. (1999). Scientizing and routinizing the assessment of suicidality in outpatient practice. *Professional Psychology: Research and Practice, 30*(5), 447–453.

Kaduson, H. G., & Schaefer, C. E. (2000). *Short-term play therapy for children.* New York: Guilford.

Kazdin, A. E. (1997). Parent management training: Evidence, outcome, and issues. *Journal of American Child and Adolescent Psychiatry, 36,* 1349–1356.

Kazdin, A. E. (1998). Psychosocial treatments for conduct disorder in children. In P. E. Nathan & J. M. Gorman (Eds.), *A guide to treatments that work* (pp. 65–89). New York: Oxford University Press.

Kazdin, A. E. (2000). Treatments for aggressive and antisocial children. *Juvenile Violence, 9,* 841–858.

Keller, M. B., McCullough, J. P., Klein, D. N., Arnow, B., Dunner, D. L., Gelenberg, A. J., et al. (2000). A comparison of nefazodone, the cognitive behavioral-analysis system of psychotherapy, and their combination for the treatment of chronic depression. *New England Journal of Medicine, 342,* 1462–1470.

Kendler, K. S., Masterson, C. C., Ungaro, R., & Davis, K. L. (1984). A family history study of schizophrenia-related personality disorders. *American Journal of Psychiatry, 141,* 424–427.

Koenigsberg, H. W., Woo-Ming, A. M., & Siever, L .J. (2002). Pharmacological treatments for personality disorders. In P. E. Nathan & J. M. Gorman (Eds.), *A guide to treatments that work* (2nd ed.; pp. 625–641). New York: Oxford University Press.

Leahy, R. L., & Holland, S. J. (2000). *Treatment plans and interventions for depression and anxiety disorders.* New York: Guilford.

Leifer, R. (1999). Buddhist conceptualization and treatment of anger. *Journal of Clinical Psychology, 55,* 339–351.

Linehan, M. M. (1993a). *Cognitive behavior therapy of borderline personality disorder.* New York: Guilford.

Linehan, M. M. (1993b). *Skills training manual for treatment of borderline personality disorder.* New York: Guilford.

Linehan, M. M., Hubert, A., Suarez, A., Douglas, A., & Heard, H. (1991). Cognitive-behavioral treatment of chronically parasuicidal borderline patients. *Archives of General Psychiatry, 48,* 1060–1064.

REFERENCES

Linehan, M. M., & Kehrer, C. A. (1993). Borderline personality disorder. In D. H. Barlow (Ed.), *Clinical handbook of psychological disorders* (2nd ed., pp. 396–441). New York: Guilford.

Longabaugh, R., & Morgenstern, J. (1999). Cognitive behavioral coping skills therapy for alcohol dependence: Current status and future directions. *Alcohol Research and Health, 23*, 78–85.

Marlatt, G. A. (1998). Basic principles and strategies of harm reduction. In A. G. Marlatt (Ed.), *Harm reduction: Pragmatic strategies for managing high-risk behaviors* (pp. 49–66). New York: Guilford.

Masterson, J. F., & Klein, R. K. (1989). *Psychotherapy of the disorders of the self.* New York: Brunner/Mazel.

Mayne, T. J., & Ambrose, T. K. (1999). Research review on anger in psychotherapy. *Journal of Clinical Psychology, 55*, 353–363.

McCullough, J. P. (2000). *Treatment for chronic depression: Cognitive behavioral analysis system of psychotherapy.* New York: Guilford.

McGinnis, E., & Goldstein, A. P. (1997). *Skillstreaming the elementary school child: New strategies and perspectives for teaching prosocial skills.* Champaign, IL: Research Press.

McMahon, R. J., & Wells, K. C. (1998). Conduct problems. In E. J. Mash & R. A. Barkley (Eds.), *Treatment of childhood disorders* (pp. 111–207). New York: Guilford.

Miller, T. W., Leukefeld, C. G., & Jefferson, B. (1996). Dual diagnosis: Clinical issues in the treatment of substance abuse, and affective, personality, and psychotic disorders. *Journal of Contemporary Psychotherapy, 26*, 73–82.

Miller, W. R. (1978). Behavioral treatment of problem drinkers: A comparative outcome study of three controlled drinking therapies. *Journal of Consulting and Clinical Psychology, 46*, 74–86.

Miller, W. R., & Rollnick, S. (1991). *Motivational interviewing: Preparing people to change addictive behavior.* New York: Guilford.

Miller, W. R., & Rollnick, S. (2002). *Motivational interviewing: Preparing people for change* (2nd ed.). New York: Guilford.

Millon, T. (1981). *Disorders of personality DSM–III: Axis II.* New York: Wiley.

Millon, T. (1993). Negativistic (passive-aggressive) personality disorder. *Journal of Personality Disorders, 7*, 79–85.

Millon, T., & Radovanov, J. (1995). Passive-aggressive (negativistic) personality disorder. In W. J. Livesley (Ed.), *The DSM–IV personality disorders: Diagnosis and treatment of mental disorders* (pp. 312–325). New York: Guilford.

Monti, P. M., & Rohsenow, D. J. (1999). Coping-skills training and cue exposure therapy in the treatment of alcoholism. *Alcohol Research and Health, 23*, 107–115.

Nadeau, K. G. (1995). *A comprehensive guide to attention deficit disorder in adults: Research, diagnosis, and treatment.* New York: Brunner/Mazel Publishers.

Nathan, P. E., & Gorman, J. M. (1998). Treatments that work—And what convinces us they do. In P. E. Nathan & J. M. Gorman (Eds.), *A guide to treatments that work* (pp. 3–25). New York: Oxford University Press.

Negy, C. (1995). Coping styles, family dynamics, and prison adjustment: An investigation of White, Black, and Hispanic offenders (Doctoral dissertation, Texas A&M University, 1995). *Dissertation Abstracts International, 55*, 4610.

Negy, C., Woods, D. J., & Carlson, R. (1997). The relationship between female inmates' coping and adjustment in a minimum-security prison. *Criminal Justice and Behavior, 24,* 224–233.

Ornstein, P. H. (1999). Conceptualization and treatment of rage in self psychology. *Journal of Clinical Psychology, 55,* 283–293.

Paivio, S. C. (1999). Experiential conceptualization and treatment of anger. *Journal of Clinical Psychology, 55,* 311–324.

Prochaska, J. O., DiClemente, C. C., & Norcross, J. C. (1997). In search of how people change: Applications to addictive behaviors. In G. A. Marlatt & G. R. VandenBos (Eds.), *Addictive behaviors: Reading on etiology, prevention, and treatment* (pp. 671–696). Washington, DC: American Psychological Association.

Pugh, D. (1993). The effects of problem-solving ability and locus of control on prisoner adjustment. *International Journal of Offender Therapy and Comparitive Criminology, 37,* 163–176.

Quay, H. C. (1986). Conduct disorders. In H. C. Quay & J. S. Werry (Eds.), *Psychopathological disorders of childhood* (3rd ed., pp. 35–72). New York: Wiley.

Reitzel, L. R., & Harju, B. L. (2000). Influence of locus of control and custody level on intake and prison-adjustment depression. *Criminal Justice and Behavior, 27,* 625–644.

Resick, P. A., & Calhoun, K. S. (2001). Post-traumatic stress disorder. In D. H. Barlow (Ed.), *Clinical handbook of psychological disorders* (3rd ed., pp. 60–114). New York: Guilford.

Robins, S., & Novaco, R. W. (1999). Systems conceptualization and treatment of anger. *Journal of Clinical Psychology, 55,* 325–337.

Roemer, L., & Orsillo, S. M. (2002). Expanding our conceptualization of and treatments for generalized anxiety disorder: Integrating mindfulness/acceptance-based approaches with existing cognitive-behavioral models. *Clinical Psychology: Science and Practice, 9,* 54–68.

Room, R. (1998). *The co-occurrence of mental disorders and addictions: Evidence on epidemiology, utilization and treatment outcomes* (ARF Research Document 141). Toronto: ARF Division, Centre for Addiction and Mental Health.

Roy-Byrne, P. P., & Cowley, D. S. (2002). Pharmacological treatments for panic disorder, generalized anxiety disorder, specific anxiety disorder, and SAD. In P. E. Nathan & J. M. Gorman (Eds.), *A guide to treatments that work* (2nd ed., pp. 337–353). New York: Oxford University Press.

Ryan, R. M., & Deci, E. L. (2000). Self-determination theory and the facilitation of intrinsic motivation, social development, and well-being. *American Psychologist, 55,* 68–78.

Schaeffer, C. E., Jacobsen, H. E., & Ghahramanlou, M. (2000). Play group therapy for social skills deficits in children. In H. G. Kaduson & C. E. Schaefer (Eds.), *Short-term play therapy for children* (pp. 296–344). New York: Guilford.

Scheel, K. R. (2000). The empirical basis of dialectical behavioral therapy: Summary, critiques, and implications. *Clinical Psychology: Science and Practice, 7,* 68–86.

Schlenker, B. R., & Leary, M. R. (1982). Social anxiety and self-presentation: A conceptualization and model. *Psychological Bulletin, 92,* 641–669.

Schneier, F. R., Johnson, J., Hornig, C. D., Liebowitz, M. R., & Weissman, M. M. (1992). Social phobia: Comorbidity and morbidity in an epidemiological sample. *Archives of General Psychiatry, 49,* 282–288.

REFERENCES

Schultz, S. C., Schultz, P. M., & Wilson, W. H. (1988). Medication treatment of schizotypal personality disorder. *Journal of Personality Disorders, 2,* 1–13.

Siever, L. J., & Kendler, K. S. (1986). Schizoid/schizotypal/paranoid personality disorders. In A. M. Cooper, A. S. Frances, & M. H. Sacks (Eds.), *Personality disorders and neuroses* (pp. 191–201). Philadelphia: J. B. Lippincott.

Slaby, R. G., & Crowley, C. G. (1977). Modification of cooperation and aggression through teacher attention to children's speech. *Journal of Experimental Child Psychology, 23,* 442–458.

Snyder, D. K. (1979). Multidimensional assessment of marital satisfaction. *Journal of Marriage and the Family, 41,* 813–823.

Snyder, K. V., Kymissis, P., & Kessler, K. (1999). Anger management for adolescents: Efficacy of brief group therapy. *Journal of the American Academy of Child and Adolescent Psychiatry, 38,* 1409–1416.

Spanier, G. B. (1976). Measuring dyadic adjustment: New scales for assessing the quality of marriage and similar dyads. *Journal of Marriage and the Family, 38,* 15–28.

Sperry, L. (1995). *Handbook of diagnosis and treatment of the DSM–IV personality disorders.* New York: Brunner/Mazel.

Sukhodolsky, D. G., Solomon, R. M., & Perine, J. (2000). Cognitive-behavioral, anger-control intervention for elementary school children: A treatment-outcome study. *Journal of Child and Adolescent Group Therapy, 10,* 159–170.

Tripp, G., & Sutherland, D. M. (1999). Counseling boys with attention-deficit/hyperactivity disorder. In A. M. Horne & M. S. Kiselica (Eds.), *Handbook of counseling boys and adolescent males: A practitioner's guide.* Thousand Oaks, CA: Sage.

Turner, R. M. (2000). Understanding dialectical behavioral therapy. *Clinical Psychology: Science and Practice, 7,* 95–98.

Wainberg, M. L., Keefe, R. S. E., & Siever, L. J. (1995). The neuropsychiatry of schizotypal personality disorder. In J. J. Ratey (Ed.), *Neuropsychiatry of personality disorders* (pp. 210–229). Cambridge, MA: Blackwell Science.

Walters, G. D. (2000). Behavioral self-control training for problem drinkers: A meta-analysis of randomized control studies. *Behavior Therapy, 31,* 135–149.

Wetzler, S., & Morey, L. C. (1999). Passive-aggressive personality disorder: The demise of a syndrome. *Psychiatry: Interpersonal and Biological Processes, 62,* 49–59.

Westen, D. (2000). The efficacy of dialectical behavioral therapy for borderline personality disorder. *Clinical Psychology: Science and Practice, 7,* 92–94.

Wettstein, R. M. (1998). *Treatment of offenders with mental disorders.* New York: Guilford.

Wheeler, J. G., Christensen, A., & Jacobson, N. S. (2001). Couple distress. In D. H. Barlow (Ed.), *Clinical handbook of psychological disorders* (pp. 609–630). New York: Guilford.

Wilson, G. T., & Fairburn, C. G. (1998). Treatments for eating disorders. In P. E. Nathan & J. M. Gorman (Eds.), *Treatments that work* (pp. 501–530). New York: Oxford University Press.

Wolpe, J., & Lazarus, A. A. (1966). *Behavior therapy techniques.* New York: Pergamon Press.

Young, J. (1987). *Schema-focused cognitive therapy for personality disorders.* Unpublished manuscript.

Young, J. E., Beck, A. T., & Weinberger, A. (1993). Depression. In D. H. Barlow (Ed.), *Clinical handbook of psychological disorders* (2nd ed., pp. 240–277). New York: Guilford.

Zuckerman, M. (1999). *Vulnerability to psychopathology: A biosocial model.* Washington, DC: American Psychological Association.

Forthcoming

A companion book, *Simple Treatment for Complex Problems: A Patient Workbook,* by Kelly C. Cukrowicz, Andrea B. Burns, Jennifer A. Minnix, Lorraine R. Reitzel, and Thomas E. Joiner, will be available in the spring of 2004. It will constitute a reader-friendly guide and set of exercises both for patients seeking to enhance skills learned in therapy sessions and for those attempting to address their problems without professional assistance.

The workbook includes an appendix detailing applications of the general techniques to specific psychological disorders and common interpersonal difficulties, and sample worksheets.

For further information or to order:

www.erlbaum.com

Order Department
Lawrence Erlbaum Associates
10 Industrial Avenue
Mahwah, NJ 07430–2262

800 926–6579   9:00–5:00 E.S.T.
201 760–3735   facsimile
orders@erlbaum.com

Author Index

A

Alberti, R. E., 21
Ambrose, T. K., 170, 171
American Psychiatric Association, 8, 10, 15, 16, 33, 34, 49, 50, 67, 81, 82, 102, 103, 104, 109, 119, 120, 140, 169, 170, 188, 190, 192, 215
Arnow, B., 2, 83, 84, 99, 125, 154
Asher, S. R., 139

B

Ballenger, J. C., 109
Barber, J., 68, 83
Barkley, R. A., 123, 124, 125, 127, 128, 129
Barlow, D. H., 81, 82, 83, 102, 103, 104, 105, 109, 115
Baucom, D. H., 154
Beck, A. T., 17, 19, 28, 35, 39, 51, 52, 59, 62, 65, 76, 82, 86, 99, 209, 215
Bellack, A., 17
Benjamin, L. S., 16, 35
Beutler, L., 68
Bloomquist, M. L, 123, 124, 125, 127, 129, 140, 141, 142
Bodholdt, R., 192
Boothby, J., 188, 189, 202, 203
Borkovec, T. D., 103, 109
Bowers, C. A., 215
Breiner, M. J., 215
Brestan, E. V., 122

Brosnan, R., 121
Brown, T. A., 82, 109, 115
Butler, G., 103, 109

C

Calhoun, K. S., 31
Carlson, R., 193
Carr, A., 121
Chambless, D. L., 2
Christensen, A., 154
Clements, C., 188, 189, 202, 203
Cohen, E. M., 81, 82, 83
Costello, E., 103, 109
Cowley, D. S., 83
Craske, M. G., 104, 105
Crits-Christoph, P., 17, 51, 68, 83
Crowley, C. G., 140

D

Dahlen, E. R., 171
Daiuto, A. D., 154
Davis, K. L., 16
Deci, E. L., 84
Deffenbacher, J. L., 170, 171
DiClemente, C. C., 215
Douglas, A., 68
Drummond, P. D., 171
Dunn, M. E., 215
Dunner, D. L., 2, 83, 84, 99, 125, 154
Dvoskin, J. A., 192

E

Ellis, A., 89
Emery, G., 36
Emmons, M. L., 21
Engel, D., 68
Esler, J. L., 102, 103, 104, 109
Estrada, A. U., 121, 126
Eyberg, S. M., 122

F

Fairburn, C. G., 216
Fennell, M., 103, 109
Fleming, G., 16, 17
Frances, A. J., 16
Freeman, A., 16, 17, 19, 28, 36, 39, 51, 52, 59, 62, 65, 76, 82, 86, 99
Friedel, R. O., 16
Fuller, R. K., 215

G

Gabbard, G. O., 16
Gacono, C. B., 192
Gelder, M., 103, 109
Gelenberg, A. J., 2, 83, 84, 99, 125, 154
Gerzina, M. A., 171
Ghahramanlou, M., 140
Goldberg, S. C., 16
Goldstein, A. P., 142
Gorman, J. M., 15, 102, 193, 209
Gowensmith, W. N., 171
Grawe, K., 68
Green, A., 33
Greenberg, L. M., 154

H

Haddock, G., 17
Hafemeister, T. L., 192
Hall, S. R., 192

Hamer, R. M., 16
Harju, B. L., 193
Heard, H., 68
Heimberg, R. G., 82, 83, 90
Hersen, M., 17
Hiller-Sturmofel, S., 215
Hollon, S. T., 209, 215
Holland, S. J., 91, 109, 111
Hope, D. A., 82, 83, 90
Hope, R. A., 216
Hornig, C. D., 82
Hoyt, R., 16
Hubert, A., 68
Hymowitz, P., 16

I

Irwin, J. E., 215

J

Jacobsberg, L. B., 16
Jacobsen, H. E., 140
Jacobson, N. S., 154
Jefferson, B., 219
Jobes, D. A., 98
Johnson, J., 82
Johnson, R. A., 219
Johnson, S. M., 154
Joiner, T. E., 50, 98
Jones, R., 216
Juster, H., 82

K

Kaduson, H. G., 140, 141, 142
Kazdin, A. E., 120, 121, 122, 123, 125, 126
Keefe, R. S. E., 16
Kehrer, C. A., 35, 37
Keller, M. B., 2, 83, 84, 99, 125, 155
Kendler, K. S., 16

AUTHOR INDEX

Kessler, K., 171
Kinney, C., 17
Klein, D. N., 2, 83, 84, 99, 125, 154
Klein, R. F., 35
Koenigsberg, H. W., 83
Kymissis, P., 171

L

Lang, A. R., 215
Lazarus, A. A., 86
Leahy, R. L., 91, 109, 111
Leary, M. R., 82
Lebow, J., 154
Leifer, R., 170
Leukefeld, C. G., 219
Liebowitz, M. R., 82
Linehan, M. M., 34, 35, 37, 38, 68, 89, 99
Longabaugh, R., 215
Lynch, R. S., 171

M

Markowitz, J. C., 2, 83, 84, 99, 125, 154
Marlatt, G. A., 215
Masterson, C. C., 16
Masterson, J. F., 35
Mayne, T. J., 170, 171
McCarthy, E., 17
McCullough, J. P., vii–viii, 2, 3, 7, 16, 39, 52,
    67, 83, 84, 86, 88, 89, 99, 101, 102, 115,
    123, 125, 127, 141, 142, 150, 154, 165,
    175, 211, 214, 220
McGinnis, E., 142
McMahon, R. J., 140
Miller, T. W., 219
Miller, W. R., 64, 98, 215, 216
Millon, T., 16, 50
Mohr, D., 68
Monti, P. M., 214
Morey, L. C., 50
Morgenstern, J., 215
Morris, C. D., 171

Mueser, K. T., 154
Munez, L., 68

N

Nadeau, K. G., 217
Nathan, P. E., 15, 102, 193, 209
Negy, C., 193
Neiberding, R. J., 192
Nemeroff, C. B., 2, 83, 84, 99, 125, 154
Norcross, J. C., 215
Novaco, R. W., 170

O

O'Connor, M., 216
O'Leary, T. A., 109, 115
Ollendick, T. H., 2
Ornstein, P. H., 170
Orsillo, S. M., 89
Owen, A., 192

P

Paivio, S. C., 174
Perine, J., 171
Pinsof, W. M., 121, 126
Pretzer, J., 16, 17
Prochaska, J. O., 215
Pugh, D., 193

Q

Quay, H. C., 119

R

Radovanov, J., 50
Raffa, S. D., 81, 82, 83
Rector, N. A., 17
Reitzel, L. R., 193

Resick, P. A., 31
Resnick, R. J., 16
Robins, S., 170
Robson, P., 103, 109
Roemer, L., 89
Rohsenow, D. J., 214
Rollnick, S., 64, 98, 215, 216
Room, R., 219
Roy-Byrne, P. P., 83
Rubel, J., 192
Rudd, M. D., 50, 98
Rush, A. J., 36
Russell, J. M., 2, 83, 84, 99, 125, 154
Ryan, R. M., 84

S

Schaefer, C. E., 140, 141, 142
Scheel, K. R., 38
Schlenker, B. R., 82
Schneier, F. R., 82
Schultz, S. C., 16
Schultz, P. M., 16
Shaw, B. F., 36
Shoham, V., 154
Sickles, M., 16
Siever, L. J., 16, 83
Simon, K. M., 16, 17
Slaby, R. G., 140
Snyder, D. K., 156
Snyder, K. V., 171
Solomon, R. M., 171
Spanier, G. B., 156
Spaulding, W., 17
Sperry, L., 16
Stickle, T. R., 154
Stritzke, W. G. K., 215
Suarez, A., 68
Sukhodolsky, D. G., 171
Sutherland, D. M., 120, 121

T

Tarrier, N., 17

Thase, M. E., 2, 83, 84, 99, 125, 154
Tripp, G., 120, 121
Trivedi, M. H., 2, 83, 84, 99, 125, 154
Turner, R. M., 38

U

Ungaro, R., 16

V

Vitali, A. E., 102, 103, 104, 109

W

Wainberg, M. L, 16
Walker, R. L., 98
Walters, G. D., 215
Wang, M. C., 215
Weinberger, A., 36
Weissman, M. M., 82
Wells, K. C., 140
Westen, D., 38
Wettstein, R. M., 204
Wetzler, S., 50
Wheeler, J. G., 154
Wilson, G. T., 216
Wilson, W. H., 16
Wolpe, J., 86
Woods, D. J., 193
Woo-Ming, A. M., 83

Y

Young, J. E., 36, 39
Yusupoff, L., 17

Z

Zajecka, M., 2, 83, 84, 99, 125, 154
Zuckerman, M., 102

Subject Index

A

Actual Outcome (AO), *see also* Situational Analysis
  definition, 5–7
Adjustment Disorder, 188–205
  active type, 190–192
  case examples, 194–202
  comorbidity, 190, 192, 198, 204
  passive type, 189–190
  treatment, 192–205
    anger management, 193
    cognitive behavioral, 193
    Cognitive Behavioral Analysis System of Psychotherapy (CBASP), 193–205
    exposure, 193
    forensic hospital setting, 197–202
    prison setting, 192–197
    treatment obstacles, 202–205
Aging, 218
Agoraphobia, 102, 108
Anger management problems, 11, 169–186, 193, 208
  case example, 180–184
  definition, 11, 170
  disorders, 169–170
  treatment, 170–186, 193
    cognitive behavioral, 170–171
    Cognitive Behavioral Analysis System of Psychotherapy (CBASP), 171–186
    group therapy, 179–184
    prison setting, 193
    relaxation training, 171, 173
    role play, 171

self-monitoring, 171
    treatment obstacles, 184–186
Anorexia, 216–217
Anxiety Disorders, 9–10, 81–115
Antisocial behavior (ASB), 120
Antisocial Personality Disorder, 170, 192, 198, 219
Attention-Deficit/Hyperactivity Disorder (ADHD), 11, 119–137, 140, 217
  case example, 132–135
  comorbidity, 120–121
  definition, 11, 119–120
  prevalence, 140
  treatment
    Cognitive Behavioral Analysis System of Psychotherapy (CBASP), 123–137, 217
    group therapy, 126–136
    Multisystemic Therapy (MST), 121–122
    Parent Management Training (PMT), 120–126
    pharmacotherapy, 120
    Problem-Solving Skills Training (PSST), 121–123
    treatment obstacles, 135–137
Avoidant Personality Disorder (APD), 8, 16–17, 82
  treatment, *see* Social Anxiety Disorder

B

Behavioral Marital Therapy (BMT), 154
Bipolar Disorder, 198, 218

240   SUBJECT INDEX

Borderline Personality Disorder (BPD),
    8–9, 33–48, 170, 198, 208–209, 221
  biosocial theory, 34
  case example, 40–46
  definition, 8–9, 33–34, 170
  dichotomous thought, 36, 39
  prevalence, 33–34
  treatment, 8, 35–48
    cognitive, 36–38
    Cognitive Behavioral Analysis System
      of Psychotherapy, 38–48
    Dialectical Behavioral Therapy, 37–38
    interpersonal approach, 35
    psychosocial, 8
    psychotherapy, 35
    schema-focused, 36–37
    treatment obstacles, 46–48
Bulimia, 216

C

Cognitive Behavioral Analysis System of
    Psychotherapy (CBASP), vii, 2–11,
    15–19, 21–32, 38–48, 52–78, 101–115,
    123–137, 142–152, 155–166, 171–186,
    193–205, 207–223
  adjustment disorders, 193–205
  aging, 218
  anger, 11, 171–186
  Anorexia, 216–217
  anxiety disorders, 10
  application to other disorders, vii, 7–8
  Attention-Deficit/Hyperactivity Dis-
    order, 123–137
  behavioral problems, 11
  Borderline Personality Disorder, 38–48
  Bulimia, 216
  components of, 3–7
    see Situational Analysis
  compulsive gambling, 216
  Conduct Disorder, 123–137
  correctional settings, 193–205
  couples, 11, 155–166

depression, chronic, vii, 2, 84, 99, 125, 220
development of, 2–3
eating disorders, 216–217
future directions, 207–223
Generalized Anxiety Disorder, 101–103,
    108–115
health psychology, 218
learning disorders, 217–218
Oppositional Defiant Disorder, 123–137
overview, vii–viii
Panic Disorder, 101–108
parents, 10
partner relational problem, 155–166
Passive-Aggressive Personality Disorder,
    52–66
Personality Disorder Not Otherwise
    Specified (PD NOS), 67–78
research implications, 220–223
Schizotypal Personality Disorder, 15–32
settings, 12
sexual addiction, 216
social skills, 141–152
Substance Abuse Disorder, 214–216
Cognitive behavioral group therapy
    (CBGT), 83, 91–91
Cognitive therapy, 17, 36–38, 51, 65, 83, 86,
    89, 102–103, 109, 170–171, 193
Conduct Disorder (CD), 11, 119–137, 140,
    169
  comorbidity, 120–121
  definition, 11, 119–120, 169
  prevalence, 140
  treatment, 120–137
    Cognitive Behavioral Analysis System
      of Psychotherapy (CBASP), 123–
      137
    group therapy, 126–136
    Multisystemic Therapy (MST), 121–
      122
    Parent Management Training (PMT),
      120–126
    Problem-Solving Skills Training
      (PSST), 121–123
    treatment obstacles, 135–137

SUBJECT INDEX **241**

Coping Survey Questionnaire (CSQ), *see* Situational Analysis

Correctional settings, 187–205, 211
  Adjustment Disorder, 188–205
    active type, 190–192
    case examples, 194–202
    comorbidity, 190, 192, 198, 204
    passive type, 189–190
    treatment, 192–205
      anger management, 193
      cognitive behavioral, 193
      Cognitive Behavioral Analysis System of Psychotherapy (CBASP), 193–205, 211
      exposure, 193
      forensic hospital setting, 197–202
      prison setting, 192–197
      treatment obstacles, 202–205

Couples, *see* Partner relational problem

D

Dependent Personality Disorder, 8, 198
Depression, chronic, vii, 2, 84, 99, 125, 220
Desired Outcome (DO), *see also* Situational Analysis
  definition, 5–7
Dialectical Behavioral Therapy (DBT), 37–38, 68, 99, 209, 221
Dichotomous thought, 36
Dissociative Identity Disorder, *see* Multiple Personality Disorder
Dyadic Adjustment Scale (DAS), 156

E

Eating disorders, 216
Elicitation phase, *see* Situational Analysis
Emotion-focused therapy (EFT), 154
Exposure treatment, 16, 82–83, 88–90, 91–92, 97–98, 102–104, 109, 193, 208–209

F

Forensic hospitals, *see* Correctional settings

G

Gambling, compulsive, 216
Generalized Anxiety Disorder (GAD), 101–115, 211
  case example, 110–114
  definition, 102, 108–109
  treatment, 101–115, 211
    behavioral, 109
    cognitive, 102, 109
    cognitive behavioral, 102–103, 109
    Cognitive Behavioral Analysis System of Psychotherapy (CBASP), 101–115, 211
    exposure, 102–103, 109
    nondirective, 109
    relaxation, 102, 109
    treatment obstacles, 114–115

H

Harm Reduction Therapy (HRT), 215
Health psychology, 218
Histrionic Personality Disorder, 8

I

Insight-Oriented Marital Therapy, 154
Integrative Behavioral Couples Therapy (IBCT), 154
Intermittent Explosive Disorder, 170
Interoceptive exposure, 104–105, 107–108

L

Learning disorders, 217–218

M

Marital Satisfaction Inventory (MSI), 156
Medication, *see* Pharmacotherapy
Motivational interviewing/enhancement, 215
Multiple Personality Disorder (MPD), 21
Multisystemic Therapy (MST), 121–122

N

Narcissistic Personality Disorder, 8, 219
Negativistic Personality Disorder, *see* Passive-Aggressive Personality Disorder

O

Obsessive-Compulsive Disorder (OCD), 2, 8
Oppositional Defiant Disorder (ODD), 11, 119–137, 140, 169
   case examples, 130–135
   comorbidity, 120–121
   definition, 11, 119–120, 169
   prevalence, 140
   treatment, 120–137
      Cognitive Behavioral Analysis System of Psychotherapy (CBASP), 123–137
      group therapy, 126–136
      Multisystemic Therapy (MST), 121–122
      Parent Management Training (PMT), 120–126
      Problem-Solving Skills Training (PSST), 121–123
      treatment obstacles, 135–137

P

Panic control treatment (PCT), 104–108
Panic Disorder (PD), 101–115, 209, 211
   case example, 105–107

definition, 102, 103
   treatment, 101–115, 211
      cognitive, 102, 104
      cognitive behavioral, 102–103
      Cognitive Behavioral Analysis System of Psychotherapy (CBASP), 101–115, 211
      exposure, 102–104
      interoceptive exposure, 104–105, 107–108
      Panic control treatment (PCT), 104–108
      relaxation, 102
      treatment obstacles, 107–108
Paranoid Personality Disorder, 8, 16
Parent Management Training (PMT), 120–137
   case examples, 130–135
   overview, 120–123
   treatment, 123–137
      Cognitive Behavioral Analysis System of Psychotherapy (CBASP), 123–126
      depression, 125
      group therapy, 126–136
      punishment, 124–125, 135–136
      reinforcement, 124–125
      social learning, 124–125, 135
      treatment obstacles, 135–137
Partner relational problem, 11, 153–166, 208
   case example, 159–164
   comorbidity, 153–154
   definition, 11, 153
   treatment, 154–166
      Behavioral Marital Therapy, 154
      Cognitive Behavioral Analysis System of Psychotherapy (CBASP), 155–166
      emotion-focused therapy, 154
      Insight-Oriented Marital Therapy, 154
      Integrative behavioral couples therapy, 154
      traditional behavioral couples therapy, 154

SUBJECT INDEX

treatment obstacles, 164–166
Passive-Aggressive Personality Disorder, 9,
49–66
definition, 9, 49–51
treatment, 51–66
case example, 54–63
cognitive, 51, 65
Cognitive Behavioral Analysis System
of Psychotherapy (CBASP), 52–66
Coping Survey Questionnaire (CSQ),
54–65
treatment obstacles, 64–66
Personality disorders, 8–9, 15–78, 219
Personality Disorder Not Otherwise
Specified (PD NOS), 9, 67–78
case example, 69–76
definition, 9, 67–68
treatment, 67–78
Cognitive Behavioral Analysis System
of Psychotherapy (CBASP), 67–78
Dialectical Behavior Therapy, 68
treatment obstacles, 76–78
Pharmacotherapy, 2, 16, 20, 30–31, 83–84,
120, 218–219
Post-Traumatic Stress Disorder (PTSD), 19,
31
Prisons, *see* Correctional settings
Problem-Solving Skills Training (PSST),
121–123
Progressive Muscle Relaxation (PMR),
173
Psychotherapy, vii–viii, 2, 16, 35
Borderline Personality Disorder, 35
chronic depression, vii, 2
treatment, vii–viii
Schizotypal Personality Disorder, 16
Psychotic Disorder Not Otherwise Speci-
fied, 198

R

Relaxation therapy, 83–84, 91–92, 102, 109,
171, 173, 209
Remediation phase, *see* Situational Analysis

S

Schema-focused therapy, 36–37
Schizoaffective Disorder, 198
Schizoid Personality Disorder, 8, 16–17
Schizophrenia, 15, 198, 218–219
Schizotypal Personality Disorder (STPD),
8–9, 15–32, 35, 208, 211, 213
case example, 19–24
definition, 8–9, 15
therapy, vii–viii, 2, 16–32, 35, 208
Cognitive Behavioral Analysis System
of Psychotherapy (CBASP), 17–19,
21–32
communication skills, 22–25
Coping Survey Questionnaire (CSQ),
18–19, 24, 26–27
cognitive, 17, 25–28
cognitive behavioral, 17
communication skills, 22–25
graded exposure, 16, 208
history, 16–18
interpersonal boundary reinforcement, 16
interventions, 16
pharmacotherapy, 16, 20, 30–31
psychodynamic approach, vii–viii, 2,
16, 35
psychoeducation, 16
psychosocial training, 16
reality testing, 16
role play, 16
social skills training, 16, 21, 208
termination, 28–29
treatment obstacles, 29–32
Sexual addiction, 216
Situational Analysis (SA), 3–8, 18–19,
24, 26–27, 39–48, 53–63, 68–78,
84–87, 89–90, 101–115, 127–137,
142–152, 156–166, 173–186,
208–210
components, 3–7
Coping Survey Questionnaire (CSQ),
3–5, 18–19, 24, 26–27, 39–48, 54–65,
68–78, 101–115, 127–137, 142–152,

244   SUBJECT INDEX

Situational Analysis: CSQ *(continued)*
156–166, 173–186, 194–205,
208–223
definition, 3–7, 8
elicitation phase, 3, 6–7, 8, 53, 84–87
remediation phase, 3, 7, 8, 53–54, 84, 86–
87, 89–90, 177–179
Social Anxiety Disorder (SAD), 81–99,
208–209
case example, 91–97
comorbidity, 82, 84, 89
definition, 81–82
prevalence, 81
treatment, 8, 82–99
cognitive, 83, 86, 99
cognitive behavioral, 82–84, 86
Cognitive Behavioral Analysis System
of Psychotherapy (CBASP), 82–99
cognitive behavioral group therapy,
83, 90–91
Dialectic Behavioral Therapy, 99
exposure, 82–83, 88–90, 91–92, 97–98,
208
pharmacotherapy, 83–84
psychosocial, 8, 82–83
relaxation technique, 83–84, 91–92
role play, 83
social skills, 83

treatment obstacles, 97–99
Social learning theory, 123–125, 135
Social Phobia, *see* Social Anxiety Disorder
(SAD)
Social skills, 139–152, 208–209
case examples, 145–149
deficits, 139–141
definition, 140
overview, 139–141
training, 140–141, 208–209
treatment, 141–152
Cognitive Behavioral Analysis System
of Psychotherapy (CBASP), 141–
152
group therapy, 141–152
token economy, 150
treatment obstacles, 149–152
Structural analysis of social behavior, 35–36
Substance Abuse Disorder (SUD), 214–216,
219
Subjective Units of Distress Scale (SUDS),
86, 89, 209, 211

T

Traditional behavioral couples therapy
(TBCT), 154